Reflexology in
Pregnancy
and Childbirth

Commissioning Editor: Claire Wilson
Development Editor: Nicola Lally
Project Manager: Elouise Ball
Design Direction: Stewart Larking
Illustration Manager: Merlyn Harvey
Illustrator: Robert Britton

Reflexology in Pregnancy and Childbirth

Denise Tiran, MSc, PGCEA, RM, RGN, ADM
Director, Expectancy Ltd, UK;
Visiting Lecturer,
University of Greenwich,
London, UK

Foreword by
Maggie Evans RM, RN, HV Cert, MSc (Complementary Therapies)

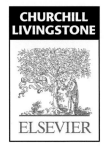

CHURCHILL LIVINGSTONE

ELSEVIER

Edinburgh London New York Oxford Philadelphia St Louis Sydney Toronto 2010

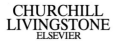

CHURCHILL
LIVINGSTONE
ELSEVIER

First published 2010, © Elsevier Limited. All rights reserved.

ISBN 978 0 7020 3110 6

British Library Cataloguing in Publication Data
A catalogue record for this book is available from the British Library

Library of Congress Cataloging in Publication Data
A catalog record for this book is available from the Library of Congress

Notice

ELSEVIER your source for books,
journals and multimedia
in the health sciences
www.elsevierhealth.com

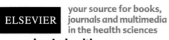

Working together to grow
libraries in developing countries
www.elsevier.com | www.bookaid.org | www.sabre.org

ELSEVIER BOOK AID International Sabre Foundation

The
Publisher's
policy is to use
**paper manufactured
from sustainable forests**

Printed in China

Contents

Contents

Foreword

It is an honour and a pleasure to be asked to write this foreword to *Reflexology in Pregnancy and Childbirth*. It is surely a most timely book when reflexology features as one of the most popular therapies to be used by midwives and complementary therapists working within maternity care. Those who are passionate about women's choices and holistic care are increasingly choosing to utilise the benefits of this ancient art.

Since time began it has been culturally acceptable to seek natural remedies and techniques to enhance women's pregnancy and birthing experiences. Tactile therapies such as massage and the use of essential oils have always been viewed as a means of nurturing the mother and her fetus to maintain a healthy pregnancy, prevent potential problems and ensure a positive birth outcome. Well over 300 years ago English midwives used sweet-smelling oils for massage in labour, whilst reflexology and acupuncture have been known to have been used for at least 3000 years, being cited in ancient Chinese texts of obstetrics. The classic Egyptian hieroglyphics displaying two practitioners with two patients appearing to be giving a foot massage treatment clearly indicates that this was regarded as a health-related therapy as it is displayed in the tomb of a well-respected physician. In the last four decades the interest and use of reflexology has escalated in line with other complementary therapy modalities, and is now gaining credibility alongside orthodox medicine.

Reflexology has a positive role to play within maternity care when due regard to safety within the context of normal midwifery or a complementary therapist's professional practice is employed. The most obvious contribution of reflexology within maternity care, as with other complementary therapies, is the potential for normalising the birth process and thus reducing the need for intervention. Reflexology provides pregnant women with an alternative choice (together with other holistic measures such as breathing techniques, self-hypnosis or aromatherapy) to help them cope better during pregnancy and childbirth. Dennis Walsh says of complementary therapies that "This [complementary therapies] resonates with physiological childbirth as a state of health and a powerful expression of wellbeing". Reflexology can be used simply to maintain that expression of wellbeing by using relaxation sequences to enhance and balance a woman's energies during pregnancy or it can be used more specifically to treat common ailments or trigger the production of endorphins and hormones to aid pain relief and assist with coping strategies during labour. When practised responsibly, reflexology can be a powerful and useful adjunct to routine normal care and can only enhance wellbeing.

Over time the observation, research and experience of renowned teachers and practitioners advances the knowledge base and understanding of therapeutic modalities. And so it is with reflexology/reflex zone therapy, evolving from early Eastern beginnings with various modifications and sub-divisions along the way to the current inclusion of reflexology into many diverse clinical and complementary settings. Several different models of reflexology now co-exist, whose facilitators have challenged core practices and philosophy. Denise stands out as such a teacher who succeeds in advancing the practice, knowledge and understanding of using reflexology within pregnancy and childbirth.

Throughout the book the incorporation of traditional reflex zone therapy techniques are fundamental to the text and a comprehensive holistic format is used by "asking, looking, listening, palpation"(which corresponds very much to an Eastern stance towards diagnosis and treatment). As in previous publications, Denise skilfully manages to employ an integrated approach, nurturing the essence of the practice and philosophy of the subject, yet weaving in the necessary precautions and evidence-based information that is pertinent to orthodox practice. However, with art and science there is also the scope to explore alternative methods and techniques, to transcend convention and to question irrational theories, especially when the underlying theory and methodology is well researched after years of practice by an informed expert. The end result is a new paradigm that cuts through traditional thoughts and theories to provide an enlightened reframing of conventional practice.

Denise is to be congratulated on her extensive knowledge and experience of reflex zone therapy which underpins her unique development of structural reflex zone therapy – a new concept in which imbalances within the musculoskeletal system are corrected via the bones in the foot. These form the reflex zones for the skeletal system, with particular attention attributed to the spinal reflexes. The theory behind this approach is based upon osteopathic principles whereby misalignment within the skeleton leads to physiological and psychological ill-health. Using traditional reflex zone therapy in tandem with structural reflex zone therapy results in innovative and succinct techniques that can be facilitated within a busy maternity unit where the luxury of time is often not available. Whilst this may be viewed by some as reductionist in its approach, there is also the need to establish "new ways of doing" when conventional practice (such as insistence on performing a full reflexology treatment for example) is too limiting or time-consuming.

As with any subject, moving from novice to expert takes time and commitment. The key to this journey lies within this book as Denise imparts her wealth of knowledge to midwives and therapists who wish to give effective and safe reflexology treatment to women during pregnancy and childbirth. *Reflexology for Pregnancy and Childbirth* is an enlightening and powerful book that is destined to lead the way forward for those midwives and therapists who share a passion for reflexology and motherhood.

Maggie Evans
Freelance lecturer in midwifery and complementary therapies
RM, RN, HV Cert, MSc (Complementary Therapies)

Preface

Reflexology has become increasingly popular with the general public and with pregnant women in particular. It is developing into a profession in its own right and has a growing body of research evidence to support practice. There are many different styles of reflexology around the world, with the majority being used primarily for relaxation, whilst a few have specific clinical applications and offer new tools for conventional healthcare practitioners to incorporate into their existing practice.

This book takes a *reflex zone therapy* approach, which is a variation on generic reflexology, used in orthodox healthcare, notably by midwives. It also introduces the concept of *structural reflex zone therapy*, an adaptation of reflex zone therapy devised by the author, in which the reflex zones of the feet act as a medium via which musculoskeletal misalignments of the body may be corrected. *Reflexology in Pregnancy and Childbirth* is aimed at qualified and student midwives and reflexologists, other maternity care providers such as doulas and antenatal educators, and complementary therapists from other disciplines with an interest in maternity care.

The book offers an introduction to the subject of reflexology and, specifically, to structural reflex zone therapy, including a revision of the zones and points on the feet which are used in treatment and of its application to the care of pregnant, childbearing and newly delivered mothers. The focus is essentially one of safety, professional accountability and evidence-based practice. It is not intended as a "how-to-do-it" text, as it would be inappropriate to learn a manual therapy from a book, and a formulaic approach to treatment would undermine the individualised, holistic element which is so much a feature of both complementary therapies and midwifery care. However, some suggestions for treating women with particular conditions in pregnancy, labour and the puerperium are given in the context of structural reflex zone therapy and the relevant physiology. The range of conditions explored is not exhaustive as it is hoped that this book will provide a model by which practitioners working at an advanced theoretical and practical level can rationalise for themselves the required techniques and precautions to the treatment of individual mothers.

Denise Tiran

Acknowledgements

I would like to thank Claire Wilson at Elsevier for giving me the opportunity to write this book, and for her unfailing support, both with this and numerous other projects. Thanks must go to all the mothers in south London – almost 5000 of them over the course of more than 20 years' reflexology practice – who have so willingly offered their feet for treatment and from whom I have learned so much about this intriguing therapy. I am grateful also to all the midwives who have joined me in learning more about reflex zone therapy in maternity care, especially my friends and colleagues at Queen Mary's Hospital in Sidcup, Kent, and numerous others around the country who have been kind enough to invite me to initiate them into this fascinating therapy.

I am particularly indebted to Clive O'Hara, a well-respected reflexology authority, who reviewed the original proposal for this book and gave me some insightful recommendations, but who, sadly, did not live to see its publication. The world of reflexology will be a sadder place without him.

My partner, Harry, has once again been a pillar of strength and support and I thank him particularly for all the help with relating physiology theory to reflexology practice. Most of all – as always – my love and thanks to my son, Adam, who helped with the proof-reading and with compilation of the glossary of terms. I've missed having him around whilst writing the book, but our love for, and pride in, each other has shone through many of those long (and expensive) telephone calls to Africa during his gap year. I wish him well as he embarks on his university life back in London.

Denise Tiran
London, 2009

Theoretical background to structural reflex zone therapy

1

INTRODUCTION TO REFLEXOLOGY

"Reflexology" is a generic term denoting a system of complementary healthcare which is based on the principle that one small area of the body represents a "map" or chart of the whole. It is both a new science, having an emerging physiological basis to underpin it, and an art, encompassing creativity, sensitivity and holism. Reflexology is becoming increasingly popular in the Western world, not least because of its nurturing approach. It is a form of touch therapy, in common with massage, aromatherapy, shiatsu and others, yet it is not simply foot "massage" – it has its own theories, mechanisms of action, effects, contraindications and precautions, as well as a developing body of research evidence. Together with other touch therapies, reflexology is slowly being integrated into some aspects of mainstream, conventional healthcare, such as cancer and palliative care, and multiple sclerosis and learning disability care (Bull 2007, Kohara et al 2004, Magill & Berenson 2008, Wang et al 2008, Wilkinson et al 2008). In maternity care, mothers are enjoying its relaxation effects and finding that it can be beneficial for helping them to cope with various pregnancy-related symptoms, and midwives and therapists are responding to this by developing the skills to use reflexology and touch therapies safely for expectant and childbearing women (Field et al 2008a, McNeill et al 2006, Mollart 2003).

Reflexology as a therapeutic modality is derived from ancient Chinese, Indian and Egyptian techniques, and was used in Europe as far back as the

14th century. In Russia the therapy was introduced by a neuro-psychiatrist, Dr Bekhterev, in the late 19th century, whilst in Germany the personal experience in 1890 of Dr Alfons Cornelius, recovering from illness, revealed that pressure, applied only to parts of the body which were painful, encouraged recovery more quickly than massage of the entire body. At about the same time, modern reflexology began to evolve from the observations of the American ear, nose and throat surgeon William Fitzgerald, who noticed that patients would frequently subconsciously apply pressure to their hands in an attempt to suppress pain. He discovered that native American Indians used a health system which focused on massaging the feet for relaxation and to ease pain. Fitzgerald harnessed this principle of "zone analgesia" to perform minor ear, nose and throat surgery without local anaesthesia and then investigated widely in order to define the "maps" of the reflex zones on the feet and hands. Fitzgerald and his colleagues, notably Dr Edwin Bowers and Dr Joseph Shelby Riley, refined the practice and theory of the therapy, added horizontal delineations and produced the first chart of reflex zones. Further development in the USA by the masseuse Eunice Ingham resulted in the production of the first of the modern reflexology charts and a change of name to "reflexology", while in 1950s Germany the nurse and midwife Hanne Marquardt further refined the reflex zone concept. Although reflex zone therapy (RZT) is a form of reflexology which can be used in various clinical specialist areas (see below), it has been used extensively in European midwifery practice, notably in Germany and Switzerland.

In the 21st century, UK reflexology has been classified as a "supportive" therapy in Group 2 of the House of Lords report (2000). This implies that reflexology should not normally be used in isolation but is helpful as an adjunct to other complementary therapies or to conventional healthcare. However, reflexology is more than simply a relaxation therapy and can be a very powerful therapeutic intervention in its own right. There has latterly been a move towards federal regulation within complementary therapies, instigated by the Prince of Wales' Foundation for Integrated Health following government directives for regulation of all health professionals as a result of the Shipman enquiry (O'Hara 2007). Reflexology as a generic therapy profession is gradually progressing towards voluntary self-regulation under the auspices of the Reflexology Forum, with a common core curriculum and accreditation of training establishments for pre-registration education, a requirement for continuing professional development and the establishment of codes of conduct. In January 2009 the Complementary and Natural Healthcare Council (CNHC) became the voluntary regulator for complementary therapies following a long period of consultation in association with the Prince of Wales' Foundation and with the support of the Department of Health. Its key objective is to encourage the use of complementary therapies as a "uniquely positive, safe and effective experience" (see www.cnhc. org), although Edzard Ernst, Professor of Complementary Medicine at Peninsula Medical School, believes it does not go far enough to protect the public (*The Guardian* 21st January 2009). (See References and resources section.)

Reflexology aims to engage the body's own self-healing processes, treating the whole person, i.e. the body, mind and spirit. Unlike conventional medicine, but in common with other complementary therapies, reflexology does not merely suppress the symptoms but intends to limit the adverse effects of disease or disorder, working with, rather than against, altered physiology. The function of the therapist is to act as a conduit to encourage the body to become receptive to self-healing through a focused ability to "read" and interpret the clues presented by the feet, taking into account every factor which contributes to the overall wellbeing of the individual, however trivial they may seem. To a certain extent it can be likened to learning a new language to assist in the process of restoring and maintaining homeostasis. It is claimed that reflexology is relaxing and de-stressing, relieves pain and inflammation, aids circulation and excretory processes, promotes muscle tone and balances the nervous system (Crane 1997:xii) and much of this has been verified, at least in part, by contemporary research (see Evidence base, below).

There are many theories about the mechanisms of action of reflexology. In conventional medicine the term "reflex" implies an involuntary and unconscious response to a stimulus. Reflexology aims to treat through "stimulation" of reflex points or zones on one small area of the body which appear to link involuntarily to others via an, as yet unproven, network of channels, neurones or transmitters. This "stimulation" via pressure or palpation of points on a part of the body, which represents a micro-system of the whole, aims to rebalance and maintain homeostasis, to assist in achieving physical, emotional and spiritual wellbeing. Most commonly the feet are used as this micro-system so that, through manual manipulation, distal areas of the body can be treated, since "stimulation" is reflected back from precise points – or zones – on the feet to corresponding organs or tissues. Reflexology can also be performed on the hands, tongue, face or back. Similarly, auricular acupressure focuses on the ear as a micro-system, whilst in iridology the irises of the eyes are used as the "map" which provides a tool to aid diagnosis, although iridology is not a therapeutic intervention in its own right. It should be noted, however, that in RZT (as opposed to generic reflexology) "stimulation" is only one of a range of treatment techniques; in some situations sedation or other techniques may be used to effect resolution of a particular problem. In structural RZT, manipulation is a significant feature of treatment, focusing specifically on the reflex zones for the musculoskeletal system (see Structural RZT, below).

Several theories about the mechanism of action relate to the *general concept of touch*, such as the relaxation factor induced by the release of endorphins and encephalins and the analgesic effect of manual pressure (Bender et al 2007). Touch, mainly in the form of therapeutic massage, has been shown to reduce the levels of the stress hormones, cortisol and noradrenaline (norepinephrine), and increase the "feel good factors", serotonin and dopamine (Field et al 2002, 2005, 2008, Hernandez-Rief et al 1999, McNabb et al 2006), effectively reducing stress, aiding relaxation and inducing sleep. The effects of touch on pain have been demonstrated in a number of studies: massage has been shown to lower the duration and intensity of phantom limb pain in amputees (Brown & Lido 2008), headache (Moraska & Chandler 2008), post-exercise pain (Frey Law et al 2008) and muscle fatigue (Ogai et al 2008). However, reflexology is distinctly different from massage, in that it also attempts to stimulate internal body organs and can be classified as a somatic therapy (working from inside–outwards), whereas massage generally facilitates topical relief of muscular and joint pains (working from outside–inwards).

Each foot has more than 7200 nerve endings, which interconnect with the central nervous system, enabling us to feel pain and pressure, hot and cold sensations, etc. Early theories about the mechanism of action focused on the belief that these nerve endings could be "stimulated" by manual pressure from the therapist, indirectly linking with other areas of the body and there-fore facilitating wellbeing and health through a fine-tuning of this sensory apparatus and its neural pathways. Furthermore, since stress patterns are also thought to manifest on the feet, disruption of these patterns with reflexology stimulation essentially relieves general stress, although there is no evidence supporting the notion that specific points on the feet link directly to the named body part, according to the "map". For example, why should pressure applied to the big toe relate specifically to the head and neck, as opposed merely to inducing a general sense of relaxation?

The skin contains different types of sensory nerve receptors, connected to sensory nerve endings (corpuscles) which make the feet sensitive to pressure and movement. Fine touch and slow vibration stimulate Meissner's corpuscles, situated about 0.7 mm below the surface of hairless skin; mild pressure stimu-lates tactile cutaneous mechanoreceptors, situated superficially in the epider-mis, and Ruffini mechanoreceptors in the middle of the epidermis. Stronger pressure and fast vibration stimulate Pacinian corpuscles, found at a deeper level within the dermis, as well as in subcutaneous layers, joints, periosteum and some viscera. Pressure or touch causes the cells to emit an electrical current (an "action potential"), which is carried to the brain via sensory nerves, then to local muscles for a response. The type of nerve fibre involved and the speed of transmission depend on the stimulatory effect, e.g. touch, pressure, variations in temperature and types of receptors or nerves. It has hitherto been difficult to measure objectively the manual force applied via RZT or to identify the exact physiological basis of the therapy (Tiran and Chummun 2005). However, contemporary work suggests that it may become feasible to record, via special technical apparatus, the impulses of specific skin receptors and thereby to identify the precise physiological pathways by which these impulses become effective (Asamura et al 1998, Ascari et al 2007, Makina & Shinoda 2004).

The mechanism of action has also been attributed to the *placebo effect* and to the *therapeutic relationship* between client and therapist, although both touch and the placebo effect are common to other manual therapies and are not exclusive to reflexology. The fact that the majority of clients leave a treatment session with their preconceived expectations met or even exceeded, feeling relaxed, refreshed and nurtured may contribute to its current popularity, although this does not explain the apparent success of reflexology in treating specific conditions. Evidence to demonstrate the scientific merit of reflexology is limited and the majority of studies are neither randomised, nor controlled. Further, trials in which "sham" reflexology or foot "massage" is used as a placebo arm of a study do not adequately address the potential for a therapeutic effect from the touch aspect alone. Numerous investigations of both complementary and conventional medicine demonstrate that some benefit can be obtained from any intervention, irrespective of its true therapeutic intent, suggesting that reflexology studies require a control group in which the subjects receive *no* treatment, in order to assess the true placebo effect (Ernst & Resch 1995, Meissner et al 2007). In addition, reflexology clients frequently exhibit or report signs and symptoms which appear to be responses to treatment, either during or after the session, including some reactions which do not normally occur with massage or other touch therapies (see Chapter 2, Reactions to treatment).

RZT is thought to be a combination of reflex signs, referred pain and trigger points. Referred pain occurs in an area of the body distal to the affected area, for example pain in the arm following angina pectoris or myocardial infarction. This concept was first described in the late 19th and early 20th centuries, notably by the neurologist Sir Henry Head, who recognised the reflex signs of disease, in which any internal dysfunction can be observed externally. He believed that, as internal organs do not have a comprehensive pain receptor system, impaired organs are unable to transmit pain impulses to conscious areas of the brain, but instead transmit messages to related skin (dermatomes), subcutaneous tissues and muscles in the related spinal segments, which cause either increased or decreased sensitivity to pain. A dermatome is an area of skin supplied by a spinal nerve, within a specific segment (level) of the spinal cord. Nerve impulses convey messages from the skin to the organs and vice versa, as well as between organs. Disease or disorder of an organ results in changes within the autonomic nervous system, sometimes producing pain at a point distal to the affected organ, as with shoulder pain in the case of gall bladder pathology. Conversely, dermal stimulation results in the unconscious transmission of impulses to internal organs via the afferent nerves. In the presence of pathological conditions, reflex signs arise, mediated via the autonomic nervous system, for example changes in the skin, subcutaneous tissues, muscles, joints and visceral organs. In RZT it is believed that additional reflex signs of disordered physiology can be found on the feet (using the map corresponding to the whole body), and that relevant foot zones will elicit autonomic nervous responses (reactions to treatment) in the event of related pathology, although these processes are not fully understood and have not been demonstrated in formal research studies.

Trigger points are specific hyperirritable points in skeletal muscle, associated with palpable nodules in taut bands of muscle fibres. On pressing the skin these points become sensitive to pressure, via kinetic chains, known to involve groups of muscles mobilised in complex movements of the body (Lavelle et al 2007). An example of this from conventional medicine would be the skin electrodes that detect changes in heart muscle during electrocardiogram. An active trigger point actively refers pain elsewhere in the body along nerve pathways. A latent trigger point does not yet actively refer pain, but as they influence muscle activation patterns, it may result in reduced muscle coordination and balance.

Spasm and pain in a muscle occur as a result of local or distant noxious stimuli, consequently stimulating a myofascial trigger point in the spine, leading to the formation of painful secondary trigger points. These, in turn, radiate further to more distal trigger points – arguably located as far distant from the original causative point as the soles or dorsum of the feet. This *neural pathway relationship theory* (Baldry 2005) is based on the activation, when disease develops, of peripheral nerve receptors (nociceptors) in the skin and in muscle, which send pain impulses to the brain. It was originally identified through the work of Kellgren in the late 1930s (Kellgren 1938, 1939), in which intramuscular hypertonic saline produced pain distal to the site of injection, initially thought to follow a spinal segmental pattern (Travell & Simons 1992), although this has now been disputed. Stimulation of cutaneous and subcutaneous mechano-thermal nociceptors has since been shown to eliminate the pain by activating encephalinergic inhibitory interneurons in the dorsal horn (Luo & Wang 2008, Soloman 2002), along the lines of the "gate control" theory of pain relief originally discovered by Melzack and Wall (1965).

It is considered that biological rhythms and physical and emotional wellbeing depend on an interaction between the body's electrical brainwave system and weak electromagnetic fields generated by the earth, known as *Schumann resonance* (Rubik 2002). This has prompted the theory that altered alpha brainwave activity arising from ill health may cause dissonance in the balance of electrical wave transmission from the ground to the brain to equalise the wave length. This is thought to result in congestion in the feet which affects their ability to transmit energy from the ground (Laurence et al 2000, Osman 2000), and that reflexology, in common with acupuncture, may improve the body's electromagnetic energy balance (Popp 2008). In reflexology it is thought that this can be achieved via a "sympathetic resonance" of energy exchange between the recipient and the therapist; measurable energy is conducted from the therapist, who is deemed to be healthy with a normal energy level, to the client whose compromised health results in a lower energy level, until a homeostatic balance is achieved (Zhang 1995). Conversely, if a practitioner insists on treating a client when she feels tired or unwell it is likely that she may feel refreshed at the end of the session, yet the client may feel no better, the energy transfer in this case being reversed.

There is also the suggestion of a relationship of points on the feet to the *meridians of acupuncture* (Sugiura et al 2007), which forms the basis for chi, Five Element and meridian reflexology (see below). Although not all forms of reflexology subscribe to this theory, there is growing evidence to suggest a correlation between reflexology points and acupuncture tsubos. It was stated, as long ago as 500BC in *The Yellow Emperor's Classic* textbook of internal medicine (Veith 2002), that wherever there is a painful spot on the body an acupuncture point is located, although a study by Janovsky et al (2000) appeared to refute this. In reflexology, too, pain occurs in a foot reflex point when there is actual, impending or previous pathology. It has been suggested that systemic healing is achieved by treating the relevant reflex point, distal stimulation being transmitted via the extracellular matrix throughout the whole body. Given the evolving evidence for the relationship between trigger points and acupuncture tsubos (Birch 2003, Kao et al 2006) and the "neuromodulation" – neurological stimulation – which can be achieved by inserting acupuncture needles at points distal to the affected area (Dung et al 2004: 5), this theory warrants continuing exploration. However, it is not the purpose of this book on RZT to debate in depth the possible links between contemporary generic reflexology and Eastern meridians, although digital stimulation of three specific acupuncture points on the feet and lower legs is incorporated into the clinical suggestions for intrapartum reflex zone treatment. Readers are referred to the references and resources section for further sources of information if the meridian approach is of particular interest.

TYPES OF REFLEXOLOGY

There are various styles of reflexology, mostly evolved from the same basic principles, but now contributing to the development of reflexology as a complete profession, within which there is a range of specialist areas. Variations between the charts used by practitioners of the different systems have provoked considerable contemporary professional debate (O'Hara 2002) and, to date, there is still no consensus of opinion.

Generic reflexology, as viewed by the general public and the conventional healthcare professions, is considered to be primarily a relaxation therapy involving a special form of foot massage in order to relax and energise and thereby to restore homeostasis. The majority of reflexology schools adhere to the Ingham method™, based on the original work of Eunice Ingham and her nephew, Dwight Byers, in America, using techniques which were formerly termed "compression massage of the feet". Many consumers initially find the concept of points on the feet linking to other parts of the body difficult to comprehend, although they usually appreciate the idea that rubbing the feet stimulates the circulation and aids relaxation. Many definitions of reflexology found during an internet search continue to use the word "massage", although several specify that treatment is conducted without oils or creams which are normally required for massage to prevent friction from skin-to-skin contact. Reflexology is natural and non-invasive, although not without some risks (see Chapter 2 for contraindications, precautions and reactions to treatment) and can be performed anywhere without the need for any special equipment.

Precision reflexology builds on generic reflexology and uses a process known as "linking", in which two or even three reflexology points are held simultaneously to enhance the overall impact of the treatment. During this process the practitioner is sensitive to communication from the feet so that the treatment can be precisely applied to the individual, and stimulates identified reflexes in order to connect them, linking the energy between them. A simple example of this "linking" can be found on precise points on the thumb and middle finger of each hand, located about a quarter of an inch down from the tip: pressing both together induces a tingling, pulsing or warm sensation at these two points (see Williamson 1998).

Vertical reflexology, adapted by Lynne Booth from the Ingham method™ (which is sometimes referred to as the Booth method of vertical reflexology), uses the dorsal reflex points of both hands and feet to treat clients whilst in a weight-bearing position. Initially this appears to negate the principles of generic reflexology in that many of the reflex points are located on the plantar surface (soles) of the feet. However, this method apparently enhances the ongoing effects of conventional reflexology treatment, because the body is more responsive to healing and energetic stimulation when treated briefly in a standing (upright) position. It is claimed that treating clients whilst standing enables stimulation of deeper reflex points, including possibly some which are not accessed via conventional reflexology, enabling therapeutic effects in a shorter period of time. Although originally used primarily for orthopaedic patients and following sports injury, it has been shown to be particularly useful for patients in hospices who may be less able to tolerate a long treatment (Booth 2001, 2007). Vertical reflexology also incorporates *synergistic reflexology* in which the hand and foot are worked simultaneously, concomitant working of several points as in precision reflexology and utilising newly discovered zonal trigger reflexes on the ankles.

As already mentioned, some styles, such as *reflexology-meridian therapy*, *Five Element* and an Australian version developed by Moss Arnold, *chi reflexology*, are based on the meridians of traditional Chinese medicine (TCM), in which it is thought that the body has energy channels (meridians) transporting the person's "life force" (*Qi* - pronounced "*chee*"), linking one part of the body to others, thus contributing to the "whole". In TCM there are 12 major meridians and 365 minor meridians with focus points along them, called acupoints or tsubos. It is thought that there are over 2000 tsubos, although in contemporary TCM only about 200 are commonly used. When the person is in a true homeostatic state, the *Qi* flows unimpeded, but disease, disorder or injury cause either blockages or excesses of energy at one or more of the tsubos. In TCM, acupuncture is often used to rebalance these energy variations, or moxibustion, cupping, tuina massage or acupressure may be used. In Eastern styles of reflexology, specific manual pressure techniques are employed to rebalance the *Qi* by working on the six meridians in the feet, thought to penetrate the major organs of the body. A Japanese form of reflexology, *Zoku shin do*, is thought to be over 5000 years old and is based on the Eastern idea that the foot is essential to yin–yang harmony or balance. *Vacuflex reflexology*™ involves a two-phase treatment that combines meridian rebalancing and reflex point stimulation via suction boots on the feet and suction cups on other parts of the body attached to a suction pump.

The *Advanced Reflexology Technique (ART™)* devised by Tony Porter focuses on the precise *texture* of reflex points (as opposed to discomfort felt by the client), and is based partly on the theory that many conditions have an endocrinological aetiology. Pressure applied to the feet is deeper than in many other styles of reflexology, without overwhelming the client's tolerance threshold. A special treatment sequence is used, some of the traditional techniques used in other forms are omitted or adapted and a special lubricant is applied, resulting in a treatment said to be more flowing and dynamic. However, the pressure applied in ART™ is less than the very firm pressure of the Taiwanese *Rwo Shur*, popular throughout Asia, in which treatment is applied using not only the hands but also wooden or plastic bars and a special cream to reduce friction. Conversely, in *Morrell reflex touch* an extremely light touch is used to activate both neurological and energy pathways. It was devised by Patricia Morrell, who used it effectively to relieve pain, lower blood pressure and reduce the length of hospital stay for orthopaedic patients in one of the hospitals in Cardiff, Wales (see www.morrellreflextouch.co.uk). Similarly the more contemporary *Gentle Touch Reflexology*™ is based on a belief, similar to that in homeopathy, that the more gentle (or "dilute") the application, the more powerful it becomes (see Ricks 2001). However, these types of reflexology do not adequately correlate with the theories about the physiological impact of touch and the receptors which are stimulated by different depths of pressure, thus reaffirming the theory that reflexology is more than simply a touch therapy.

Several styles of reflexology combine zone and point work with aspects of other therapies, for example *SMART Ayurvedic Reflexology* – the Stathis Method of Ayurvedic Reflex Therapy (SMART), which is a blend of the reflex maps of foot reflexology and Ayurveda's Paddabyhanga foot massage routine, using oils selected according to the individual's energy balance. Ayurvedic reflexology also uses a small metal bowl or *kansa* which is oiled and rubbed on the soles of the feet, producing heat to balance the foot and body temperatures. This is followed by stimulation of the acupuncture points in the feet to restore energetic flow, together with rose or sandalwood oils to cleanse and restore homeostasis. Other styles are emerging in which the reflexology maps of the feet are used as a medium through which to apply different therapeutic interventions, as in *foot-applied Bowen therapy. No hands reflexology*™ was devised by Gerry Pyves in response to the repetitive strain-type injury he sustained and involves the use of the elbows as a means of protecting the joints in the hands of the practitioner. *Coordinative reflexology*, an Israeli therapy devised in the 1980s, incorporates a series of flowing techniques similar to

---

Box 1.1 Types of reflexology

- Advanced reflexology technique (ART™)
- Chi reflexology
- Coordinative reflexology
- Foot-applied Bowen therapy
- Five Element reflexology
- Generic reflexology
- Gentle Touch™ reflexology
- Integrative reflexology
- Metamorphic technique
- Morell reflexology
- No hands reflexology™
- Precision reflexology
- Reflexology meridian therapy
- Reflex zone therapy/reflexotherapy
- Rwo Shur method
- SMART Ayurvedic reflexology
- Spinal reflexology
- Structural reflex zone therapy (Tiran)
- Synergistic reflexology
- Vacuflex™ reflexology
- Vertical/upright reflexology
- Zoku shin do

dance and may involve treatment being given by one or two practitioners. *Integrative reflexology* encompasses the zones and reflex points of traditional reflexology, as well as the inter-relationships linked by the body's meridians and proprioceptors, together with structural alignment techniques based on the manual therapy of rolfing.

The *Metamorphic technique*, an off-shoot of reflex zone therapy (see below), primarily focuses on the foot zones corresponding to the spine, along the inner edge of each foot. It is considered that this area reflects also a time period related to the 9 months of intrauterine life; treatment aims to correct imbalances thought to be caused by activities occurring both before and immediately after birth, and the therapy appears to have been used successfully with children with Down's syndrome and with autism (Reeson 2006). In a similar manner, *spinal reflexology* acknowledges the neurological link between the spinal vertebrae and specific nerves, organs, muscles, etc., but in this method the therapist uses the hands and thumbs on the client's back to identify which vertebrae are out of balance so that both the affected organ(s) and the nerves that serve the organ are treated. Treatment aims to "fine tune" the 31 pairs of cervical and spinal reflexes by working simultaneously on the appropriate spinal vertebrae and the corresponding organ reflex on the hand or foot (whole body reflexology).

REFLEX ZONE THERAPY

RZT (or the more contemporary term "reflexotherapy of the feet") expands on the basic tenets of generic reflexology. However, unlike some other forms, in RZT the body is divided into ten equal vertical zones and three transverse zones, demarcated by imaginary lines which correspond to transverse planes in the body. Therapists refer to a chart which differs from those used in many other types of reflexology, in which the feet are divided into ten longitudinal zones dividing the body lengthwise, with five zones on each side of the midline, and three transverse zones dividing the body horizontally, with each section corresponding to a horizontally differentiated area of the body. Zone 1 on each side of the body is in the medial aspect, and zone 5 is distal to the midline; zone 1 ends in the thumbs and big toes, whilst zone 5 ends in the little fingers and little toes.

In practical terms, RZT practitioners view the shape of the feet as similar to that of the whole body, when a person is seated in the upright position, i.e. if an individual sits with her feet up in front of her she is essentially looking at herself in a mirror. This simplifies and makes logical the location of reflex areas, the dorsum of each foot representing the front of the body, the soles being related to the internal organs and the inner and outer edges of the feet corresponding to the inner and outer aspects of the whole body respectively. The transverse zones of the feet conveniently reflect the zones for the head and neck (the toes), the thorax (the ball of the foot and the related dorsal area), the abdomen (the arch of the foot and related dorsal area) and the pelvis (the heel). The horizontal divisions correspond to the shoulder girdle at the base of the toes, the diaphragm below the ball of the foot, and the line for the pelvic brim differentiates the abdomen from the pelvis and lower body. The left foot corresponds to the left side of the body and the right foot relates to the right side of the body. Where there are two organs, such as the lungs or eyes, there is a related zone on each foot; if an organ is unilateral the reflex zone will be found only on the foot on the relevant side of the body, for example, the liver and gall bladder zones are on the right foot, whereas the spleen reflex zone is on the left. Where an organ is central but displaced to one side, such as the stomach, there will be a larger reflex zone on one foot, in this case, on the left.

In common with generic reflexology, RZT uses an approach in which physio-pathological changes within the body are reflected in one or more areas of the feet. These may be observed visually, for example, different colours, shapes, tones or textures on parts of the feet. Alternatively the practitioner may feel significant differences beneath the working fingers during manual palpation or the client may report sensations such as tenderness or energy surges in the feet, or experience systemic reactions to the treatment, both during and after the session (see Chapter 2). However, as previously stated, RZT is *not* simply a foot *massage*, although elements of massage and other therapies may be incorporated into the treatment session to aid relaxation. RZT is a *clinical modality* that aims to facilitate recognition of disordered foot zones, to relieve symptoms of physio-pathological conditions, to prevent further complications and to support the body's natural healing mechanisms. This can be achieved partly through the relaxation which is a component of all types of reflexology, and partly by working specifically on relevant points, using various manual compression techniques, some stimulating and some sedating according to the needs of the client, with the aim of re-balancing homeostasis and triggering the body's innate self-healing capacity.

The emphasis in RZT on the relating of treatment decisions to a comprehensive appreciation of the individual's physio-pathology could be said to facilitate easier incorporation into conventional *clinical practice*, as opposed to merely relaxation reflexology. Certainly, clinical RZT may work at a deeper level in that it may treat the physiological causes as well as the symptoms, although many practitioners and authorities of other types of reflexology would dispute the claim that this differs from their own modality. Conversely, this clinical approach in which the practitioner may focus treatment on the relief of specific conditions, sometimes without the accompanying "relaxation factor", could be accused by some of being more reductionist than generic reflexology, which prides itself on being "holistic", although a degree of relaxation is usually attained even with a short RZT treatment. Full training as a reflex zone therapist has hitherto been open only to students with a qualification in a conventional medical or healthcare profession, for example, midwifery, nursing, physiotherapy or osteopathy, as it requires a comprehensive

Box 1.2	Features that differentiate clinical reflex zone therapy from generic reflexology

- Based on use of ten longitudinal and three transverse zones
- More emphasis of zones on whole foot, not just the plantar surface of feet
- Clinical modality, not merely a relaxation therapy
- Variations in location of some reflex zones/charts
- Incorporates specific techniques to treat disorders – stimulation, sedation, etc.
- Focuses on treating causes not merely on alleviating symptoms

knowledge and understanding of anatomy, physiology, pathology, pharmacology and other related disciplines. However, this is changing as complementary therapy education becomes more academic.

INTRODUCING STRUCTURAL REFLEX ZONE THERAPY

Structural RZT, an adaptation of RZT devised by Tiran (2004b), builds on the zone therapy approach, in that it uses the same map of the zones (with some minor variations based on specific experience, see Chapter 3), but incorporates also an understanding of the structure and function of the body, in the same way as an osteopath views it. The theoretical basis of osteopathy is that the musculoskeletal system is the main supportive framework of the body, essentially the body's "scaffolding", with the soft tissues attached either internally or externally to the framework (although, contrary to popular opinion, osteopaths do not only treat bones, ligaments and joints, but consider the inter-relationship of *all* tissues and fluids of the body). The fundamental premise in osteopathy is that changes in anatomical structure will lead to physiological dysfunction and altered homeostasis, including chemical, neurological, electrical and biomechanical problems. Any pathological condition triggers changes in local and distal tissues, including protective muscular spasm, rebound pain and tenderness, oedema, congestion and other responses. Treating movement and musculoskeletal disharmony enables enhanced inter-communication between all parts of the body, assisting in restoring circulation and drainage of fluids, normal nerve transmission and functioning, rebalancing of the immune system and an overall return to homeostasis. However, osteopathy is not simply a system in which the body is viewed as a complex engine which can be dismantled, treated and reassembled, a criticism frequently levelled at conventional medical specialties. In keeping with other non-conventional forms of medical and healthcare practice, osteopaths consider that treatment encompasses the whole person – body, mind and spirit – rather than merely the presenting disease or disorder.

Structural RZT, like osteopathy, is based on the principal notion that structure and function are inter-related and that the body's anatomy governs physiological processes; therefore, realigning the anatomical structures of the body assists in restoring physiological homeostasis. The reflex zones on the feet, particularly those for the musculoskeletal system, are thus used as a medium through which to correct or reduce anatomical imbalances which may have contributed to physiological disorders or disease, and much more attention is given to manipulating the 26 bones in the feet (which correspond to the reflex zones for the skeletal system in the body) than in most other forms of generic reflexology.

This approach is particularly pertinent to contemporary maternity care, given that lifestyle factors impact on both physical and emotional comfort during the antenatal period, although structural RZT could also be used for other clinical specialties. Pregnancy presents most women with challenges for which they are less well prepared than they may have been prior to the mid-20th century. The pressures of modern living mean that the majority of women will have been in paid employment for some years before deciding to start a family, with, in some cases, childbearing being left until the late thirties or even the forties. There is then an expectation that conception will occur spontaneously in a short period of time, yet fertility may have been compromised by lifestyle factors such as poor diet incorporating numerous additives and preservatives, excessive carbohydrate and inadequate protein, together with excessive or inadequate exercise or prolonged use of hormonal contraceptive methods. Once conception has occurred, many women seem to expect a problem-free (i.e. *symptom*-free) pregnancy and to be able to continue to work until term with no difficulty. Many occupations involve potentially hazardous environments: continual exposure to computers or manufacturing chemicals. Even for those who do not work in paid employment, the external environment may adversely affect materno-fetal wellbeing; for example, exhaust fumes in densely urbanised areas. Periods of prolonged standing or sitting, at work, in the home or in the car, are particularly significant for maternal and fetal health, as this will compromise pelvic circulation and places undue strain on certain muscles and ligaments, whilst under-using others which would facilitate improved progress and outcome. For example, the increase in symphysis pubis discomfort and the incidence of malpositions may be attributed in part to the fact that women no longer spend time engaged in scrubbing the kitchen floor and similar activities. Furthermore, the emotional pressure of assumed social expectations can contribute to increased stress, anxiety and depression and a consequent mal-adaptation in the physical structures of the body.

The spine

It is important, in structural RZT, to have an understanding of the spinal column and the associated anatomical structures. The vertebral column consists of 24 separate vertebrae plus five fused vertebrae in the sacrum and four fused vertebrae in the coccyx, although variations may be present from birth or may develop later. The functions of the vertebrae are to support the body in an upright position, to facilitate movement and locomotion and to protect the spinal cord, through which sensory nerves travel to the brain and motor nerves travel from the brain to distal structures. Normally there are five curves within the length of the spinal column: two cervical and one each of the thoracic, lumbar and sacral curves, but these may be altered by pathological changes such as osteoporotic disease or spinal injury. Attached to the lower end of the spinal column is the bony pelvis which, in a neutral position, should give a slight anterior curve to the lumbar spine, but which increases lumbar lordosis when tilted anteriorly (as in pregnancy) or decreases it when tilted posteriorly (as in some exercises to strengthen the abdominal musculature). In utero the spine is totally flexed from the outset, and after birth the upper cervical, thoracic and sacral curves remain flexed (primary curves), whereas ongoing intrauterine and infant development cause the lower cervical and lumbar curves to develop, largely in response to walking (secondary or compensatory curves). Any major mal-adaptation occurring in the spinal column will result in its being mechanically unsound; muscle weakness or disease affecting the spinal curves leads to chronic postural defects and, consequently, poor biomechanics. Approximately two-thirds of vertebral bone is porous, spongy cancellous bone, arranged in irregular trabeculae (from the Latin for "small beams"), which are strut-like structures comprising criss-cross fibres to support the bone mass. The cancellous bone acts as a "shock absorber" and the various organisations of trabecular plates resist perpendicular compression and bending and shearing movements, as well as helping to support the weight of the body. Bone mass gradually increases throughout childhood and early adulthood, reaching its genetic peak between 20 and 40 then, in women, declining after the menopause.

The thoracic region is the area of the spine with least mobility since the function of the thoracic spine and ribs is to protect the heart, lungs and major blood vessels. However, the interaction between the thoracic, cervical and lumbar spines and the pelvic girdle means that any impairment in mobility of one section will adversely affect movement in one or more of the other sections of the spine as these are interconnected by cartilage and/or muscles. There is a natural kyphosis (curvature) of the thoracic spine which is often accentuated in women, especially as a result of weight changes, including pregnancy, enlarged breasts, such as with breast feeding or surgical enhancement, and also with the impact of lifting children, notably the habit of carrying toddlers balanced on one hip. Any lateral diversion may possibly be related to the dominance of one side of the body over the other, for example when carrying heavy loads with one hand (Middleditch & Oliver 2005:28).

The lumbar spine of five vertebrae and inter-vertebral discs presents as a posterior concave curvature (lumbar lordosis), which varies considerably according to posture and position and is greater in women in their reproductive years than in men, primarily because the hormone, relaxin, is secreted by the ovary and relaxes the spinal ligaments, symphysis pubis and sacroiliac joints. Increased weight and abdominal size, in non-pregnant as well as pregnant women, and in men, together with reduced abdominal muscle tone, will increase the lumbar lordosis, causing discomfort. Sustained inappropriate positions can also adversely affect lumbar lordosis, such as sitting (decreased lordosis) or standing (increased). Women who wear high-heeled shoes assume an altered centre of gravity, directed forwards, with a consequent increase in the pelvic tilt and lumbar lordosis. Compensatory adaptations due to misalignment of the lower limbs, or to factors such as excess weight, cause pronation of the feet and/or knees, increasing activity in the lumbar erector spinae muscle and resulting in an exaggerated lumbar lordosis. The lumbar spine articulates directly with the sacrum, therefore any change in the pelvic angle inevitably affects the lordosis. Lateral curvature of the spine (scoliosis) may be present at birth or may develop spontaneously (idiopathic) or as a functional or postural deviation. Idiopathic scoliosis is more common in girls and factors such as abnormal growth and development of the spine, laxity of the joints, curvature of the sagittal spine and neurological aspects may contribute to its presentation. Functional scoliosis may arise from muscular spasm, unequal leg length, intervertebral disc degeneration or arthritic changes. Inequality in the length of the legs is the most common cause, due to congenital irregularity, or following trauma or disease. Habitual postural adaptation can also give the appearance of differing leg lengths. The pelvis tilts on one side, the lumbar curve compensates by becoming convex on the short side and there is a corresponding convex curve in the thoracic vertebrae on the longer side.

Movement of the spine and adjacent bones, ligaments, muscles and nerves is a series of small extensions, flexions and rotations; some are unintentional and others occur as reflex actions. When movement occurs in one direction, that in another direction may be either facilitated or inhibited. Extension reduces lateral flexion and rotation; lateral flexion reduces extension and normal flexion; and rotation restricts flexion and extension. Mobility of the spine varies considerably between individuals, and may be influenced by gender, age, race, congenital factors, laxity of the ligaments and pathological disorder, as well as by height, weight, fitness and lifestyle. Adopting an habitual stance, such as pointing the chin outwards and upwards, will affect mobility of one section of the spine, in this case, the cervical vertebrae, eventually impacting lower down the spine.

The pelvic girdle is a strong framework designed to withstand major physical stresses both from the weight of the body and from force exerted when the pelvic musculature contracts. There is, of course, interdependence between the joints in the pelvis – the two sacroiliac joints, which are often asymmetrical, and the symphysis pubis – and a problem occurring in any one of them will have an impact on the other two. The sacroiliac joints transmit forces from the head, upper body and upper limbs to the lower limbs. Unusually, no muscles directly affect movement; indirect action of muscles in close proximity assists in articulation of the joints. These include mainly the erector spinae and gluteus maximus, transverse abdominis and pelvic floor muscles. Body weight is transmitted from the fifth lumbar vertebrae to the sacrum, through the sacroiliac joints, along the sacral alae and through the ischial tuberosities to the acetabulum. The sacroiliac joints also act as shock absorbers in relation to the lumbar spine. Due to the large number of ligaments, muscles and fascia connecting or crossing the spine and sacroiliac joints, any disorder in the joints will then also adversely affect the entire spine. There is an extensive nerve supply derived anteriorly from the third lumbar to the second sacral vertebrae and posteriorly from the fifth lumbar to the second sacral vertebrae. Inflammation of the joints or laxity of the local ligaments will lead to misalignment of the joint surfaces and subsequent nerve irritation, triggering referred pain in other areas such as the trunk, buttocks, leg or groin.

Structural adaptation

The physiological impact of overuse or underuse of certain parts of the body will eventually result in structural adaptation. Conditions in which there is overuse of muscles, joints and ligaments, such as repetitive strain injury – renamed by Damany and Bellis (2000) as "cumulative and constant tension complex" – usually affect small muscle groups, in this example the wrist, hand, arm and neck, although any function performed repetitively under adverse biomechanical conditions will eventually lead to muscular dysfunction. Other activities which progressively apply negative pressure and lead to musculoskeletal misalignments due to enforced adaptation in specific areas include jogging on hard surfaces, sitting at a computer, playing a musical instrument, lounging in front of the television, or merely an habitual muscle tension which results from poor posture or chronic stress. In addition increased mechanical demands on soft tissues produce abnormal fibrosity in the tissues which may contribute to structural dysfunction and musculoskeletal misalignment.

Stone (2007:6) gives a comprehensive example of a "typical patient" presenting for osteopathic treatment, in which poor posture can present with a variety of musculoskeletal misalignments, leading to complex pathological problems. For example, tilting or torsion of the head and neck can trigger headaches, eye strain, ear drainage problems leading to infections, temporomandibular pain and bite problems, dysfunction of the salivary glands and neck pain. The compensatory posture adapted in response to these discomforts causes misalignment of the shoulder girdle, which may cause thoracic tension, leading to respiratory difficulties, heartburn and hiatus hernia. Further, unilateral pelvic tilting can put tension on the renal tract, leading to residual urine in the bladder and increasing susceptibility to urinary infections; tension on the reproductive tract may lead to infertility and menstrual problems; and pelvic rotation may adversely affect the hips, knees and feet.

Underuse of parts of the body can also have adverse effects – the "use it or lose it" scenario. When tissues are immobilised for any prolonged period of time, for example following trauma or accident, or due to sedentary lifestyles, collagen fibres accumulate which attract the deposition of adipose tissue, increasing the risks of mineralisation, especially in the joints. This causes systemic rigidity and muscular contraction which restricts future movement. Smith (2005) suggests that lifelong structural dysfunction can result from several other factors. Postural and movement habits learned through imitation of parents and other learned patterns of repetitive or asymmetrical use of the body will result in unilateral conditions affecting both bony and soft tissues.

Congenital and hereditary factors may contribute to a predisposition to diseases which affect the structure and function of the body. Congenital deformities such as inequality in the length of the limbs cause the affected side of the body to be smaller than the other, and there may also be corresponding inequality between the length of the arms, an asymmetrical pelvis and slight differences between the two sides of the face (Baldry 2005:139). These variations cause the person to adopt a posture in which the weight of the body favours the shorter side, the knee on the opposite side is abducted slightly, the shoulder on the affected side slopes downwards and there is tilting of the trunk to the shorter side when walking. In another example, congenital dislocation of the hips in girls, compromises, from birth, the stability and position of the pelvis; this may cause problems later in life, including displacement of the angle of inclination of the pelvic brim, which appears to increase the tendency to fetal malposition or malpresentation in pregnancy.

Chronic stress and its systemic effects, such as insomnia, adversely affect posture, although Sarno (1998) takes a Freudian approach, believing that repressed emotion triggers muscular pain and tension, possibly due to the influence of the limbic system on the autonomic nervous and immunological systems (see also Chapter 6).

Trauma, too, will interfere with the alignment of the body as it attempts to deal with the complex guarding response required for healing. Skeletal muscles, as well as soft tissues, such as fascial and myofascial tissues, nerves and viscera, experience an inflammatory response which leads to healing but may also result in the formation of scar tissue, some of which may become keloid and which, together with the formation of internal adhesions, puts tension on surrounding tissues, reducing the range of movement. This can be likened to a square box filled with various items: if pressure is exerted on one corner of the box, the shape may change to a diamond shape, and, although the contents remain the same, their positions within the box are altered, possibly to the detriment of the whole. Another analogy is a sweater in which a pulled thread causes puckering of the material from its source to an area some way distant; the pulled thread affects both the appearance and the shape (function) of the whole sweater.

Peripheral trauma affects the central nervous system. For example, where injuries such as whiplash are involved, the neck's somatosensory system may affect control of the neck, limb, eye and respiratory muscles, as well as of some pre-ganglionic sympathetic nerves (Davis 2000). Whiplash injuries can also cause chronic pain in the neck and head, jaw fatigue and severe temporo-mandibular joint clicking (Friedman & Weisberg 2000) and may permanently affect cervical lordosis with consequent neurological tensions (Kristjansson & Jónsson 2002). A controlled study by Berglund et al (2001) identified other long-term pathological sequelae following collision impact injuries, including thoracic and lumbosacral pain, fatigue and sleep disturbance, as well as other conditions. Similarly, hypertrophy or degenerative changes, such as callous formation following clavicle or upper rib fracture, may cause compression of the related neural pathway, leading to pain, whilst changes in the angulation of these bones causes postural changes and dysfunctional breathing patterns.

Other impact trauma, such as coccygeal injury from a fall or previous limb or pelvic fractures, may also lead to musculoskeletal misalignment with tension on the surrounding muscles, joints, ligaments and nerve pathways, leading to ongoing health problems. For example, Proctor et al (2001) considered the possibility that one of the causes of dysmenorrhoea may be attributed to spinal mechanical dysfunction. Reduced spinal mobility may arise from dysfunction between the second to fourth sacral vertebrae, and between the tenth thoracic and second lumbar vertebrae, which are in close proximity to the parasympathetic and sympathetic nerve pathways for the pelvis. This can result in impairment of the sympathetic nerve supply to the blood vessels of the pelvic viscera with consequent vasoconstriction, causing menstrual pain.

In another example, the intricate link between the position of the jaw, head and vertebral column, including the lumbosacral area, implies that dental problems may impact on other links in this chain, potentially triggering musculoskeletal or organ (soft tissue) conditions, which may initially appear to be unrelated (Chinappi & Getzoff 1996). This seems to be particularly significant following fracture of the jaw or manipulation during dental surgery, as in difficult wisdom teeth extraction under general anaesthetic. Similarly, the presence of chronic dental caries can give rise to instability in the upper cervical vertebrae, leading to changes in posterior cerebral blood flow which adversely affects balance and consciousness, for example dizziness when turning the head too quickly. Any pathology in this area will trigger additional problems in the associated ligaments and joints, potentially impacting on other parts of the musculoskeletal system.

Changes in the spine and musculoskeletal system during pregnancy

During the first trimester of pregnancy, pressure from the displacement of pelvic organs by the slowly enlarging uterus causes a slight posterior rotation of the bony pelvis. Initially the bladder and pelvic floor support the increased uterine weight; later, upwards movement puts pressure on the small intestine and sigmoid colon, eventually putting additional strain on the broad ligaments supporting the uterus. The posterior rotation also affects muscular function, notably the lumbar erector spinae, hip flexors and anterior upper abdominals. Towards the end of the first trimester, as the uterus emerges from the pelvis into the abdominal cavity, the small and large intestines, stomach and liver are moved upwards, and there is tension below the diaphragm. This in turn causes extension of the lumbar spine, kyphosis of the thoracic spine and lordosis of the lower cervical spine, leading to mechanical stress at the cervico-thoracic junction (exacerbating hormonally induced nausea and vomiting due to tension on the twelfth thoracic nerve and on the vagus nerve in the neck).

In the second trimester the pelvis, which has initially rotated posteriorly, now starts to rotate anteriorly, causing further changes in the spinal curves, including increased lumbar lordosis, which puts tension on the linea alba and the anterior abdominal muscles. This may lead to tension on the xiphisternum and epigastric area (contributing to the heartburn triggered by relaxation of the cardiac sphincter), and on the pubic symphysis (leading, in some women, to symphysis pubis discomfort). The intestines no longer move upwards but instead start to distort laterally and posteriorly (resulting in a broader shape to the enlarging abdomen and an altered intestinal lumen which adds to the hormone-induced constipation experienced by many women), with stretching of the diaphragmatic ligaments, rib articulations, intercostal muscles and the fascia around the thoracic and lumbar regions.

There is an increased laxity of the ligaments in the pelvis due to additional weight and to endocrine changes, notably increased levels of relaxin and also of progesterone, making the joints more mobile and, consequently, more susceptible to strain. Hypermobility of pelvic joints is common, particularly in the third trimester when relaxin is at its highest; levels return to normal between 3 and 5 months after delivery. The unstable gait typical of a woman in late pregnancy is due mainly to the altered centre of gravity as she leans backwards to maintain equilibrium in a standing position. This causes changes in the curvature of the spinal column, particularly the classic lumbar lordosis, in which the increased weight is carried on the symphysis pubis and via the abdominal musculature; thus, the position of the head and neck alter also. Alternatively, the mother may adopt a "swayback" posture in which the pressure of the increased weight is directed behind the symphysis pubis and downwards towards the pelvic floor and pelvic ligaments, aggravating groin and perineal discomfort and laxity.

As term approaches, the relaxation of the abdominal wall causes the uterine fundus to drop downwards (engagement of the presenting fetal part). Any further expansion of the uterus occurs outwards rather than upwards, placing considerable strain on the diaphragm and epigastric region (exacerbating existing heartburn), insertion sites of the rectus abdominus muscles (possibly leading to divarification of the rectus sheath in multiparous women), stomach and other organs. Any downwards pressure affects the lower abdominal and ultimately the pelvic organs, triggering complaints such as a return to, or exacerbation of, frequency of micturition. The hormonally induced hypermobility means that the mother's side-to-side flexion remains as normal or increases, causing the uterus and abdominal cavity to rotate to the opposite side from that of the flexion (i.e. if the mother bends to the left, they are displaced to the right). In the event that the mother is unable to flex laterally or there is lack of uniformity between the two sides, this may indicate uneven mechanical balance and poor elasticity of the muscles, leading to additional strain on the ligaments and further symptomatic problems.

As the spine adapts at each stage of pregnancy, so too must the shoulder, pelvic girdle and lower limbs, and coordination between the upper and lower body is necessary to avoid pain and discomfort. Indeed, there is some change in the coordination between these planes even in women with symptom-free pregnancies, requiring considerable compensatory movement. There is an altered angle of inclination of the pelvic brim, by about 4°, whilst laxity of joints increases outwards rotation of the hips, ankles and knees, placing strain on the related muscles. The mother naturally compensates for these changes by increasing her base of gait when walking (placing the feet wider apart to form a more stable base), and applying more weight on the lateral side of the feet and on the heels (hence the tendency to dry skin around these areas). As the foot mechanics alter, corresponding soft-tissue adaptations occur, with force directed up the limbs to the hip and pelvic areas, including the muscles and ligaments in the region of the symphysis pubis, contributing to pelvic girdle instability and pain. Muscles in the abdomen and up the back will also be affected, potentially causing more discomfort. Furthermore, misaligned tension on the uterine ligaments may adversely affect expansion, positioning and function within the uterus, leading to sub-optimal fetal presentation and/ or position or an abnormal fetal lie. Other factors such as the presence of scoliosis may impact on the position of the maternal spine, also contributing to abnormal fetal positioning.

The relationship between structural reflex zone therapy and the musculoskeletal changes of pregnancy

The role of structural RZT in maternity care is to enhance the benefits of standard RZT and to build on the practitioner's understanding of the complex changes to the musculoskeletal system during the antenatal, intrapartum and puerperal periods of childbearing. Treatment is applied via the feet (and occasionally via the hands) according to the reflex zone map/chart, with some minor variations. Given that there are 26 bones in the feet, treatment with structural RZT is considerably more dynamic than standard RZT, and may include more manipulation of the feet—and certainly more than in most forms of generic reflexology used in Britain. The treatment session is usually shorter than a relaxation reflexology treatment, partly because symptoms can be effectively treated in a shorter time than is normal in generic reflexology (50 minutes to an hour). It is also important to keep treatments short because it is possible to "overdose" the mother, by using prolonged or excessively forceful manipulations of the feet (see Chapter 2, Contraindications and precautions).

In practice, treatment is a combination of the Marquardt style of RZT with some additional techniques designed to assist mothers with symptoms and complications, which may have both an endocrinological and a musculoskeletal origin, to become more comfortable and to cope with the discomforts that cannot be completely alleviated. Theoretically, decisions regarding treatment are based on an application of RZT skills to an understanding of pregnancy and childbearing physiopathology, both in conventional terms *and* with an appreciation of the impact of musculoskeletal adaptations in individual women.

THE EVIDENCE BASE FOR REFLEXOLOGY

Reflexology is a relatively new concept to those working in conventional medicine, and it is sometimes difficult to explain its effects and mechanism of action to orthodox medical practitioners, especially since the concept of *energy* is alien to many. Some complementary therapists resist the academic emphasis of contemporary practice, but it is not appropriate to become defensive when challenged by allopathic practitioners, as this does nothing to stimulate the academic and professional discussion, which is so much a part of modern healthcare science. If reflexology is to be accepted into mainstream healthcare it is vital that practitioners are aware of the research evidence to support their claims for the therapy. Even an awareness of those studies which seem to be "negative", in that they do not demonstrate that reflexology "works", contribute to the wider body of knowledge and assist in refining research methodology for future studies.

Many early reflexology published papers were case reports of apparently successful resolutions to particular problems resulting from a patient receiving reflexology, but that does not infer that the therapy was the specific palliative modality. Several more recent studies focus on the benefits of the relaxation effects, and suggest that the technique can be taught to relatives, especially in oncology care (Stephenson et al 2007). Various investigations have explored the neurohormonal implications of generic touch, such as the lowering of cortisol (Bello et al 2008, Billhult et al 2008, McNabb et al 2006), with varying results. However, a distinction should be made between reflexology, foot massage and touch, although evidence of effectiveness of reflexology is sparse compared to that for touch in general. Some single-blind studies demonstrate the possible analgesic properties of reflexology (Stephenson et al 2003), whilst others focus on the relief of anxiety, depression and stress (Lee 2006, Quattrin et al 2006) and insomnia (Song & Kim 2006), although the placebo effect and the impact of touch alone cannot be excluded.

A few studies have explored the physiological effects induced by reflexology, including the reduction of blood pressure (Park & Cho 2004), heart rate (Sugiura et al 2007) and changes in the blood flow to organs corresponding to the foot zones being stimulated, such as the intestines (Mur et al 2001) and the renal tract (Sudmeier et al 1999). Others have considered the specific effects of reflexology on symptoms and conditions, some apparently successful, such as for urinary incontinence (Mak et al 2007), chemotherapy-related nausea (Yang 2005), paediatric constipation and encopresis (Bishop et al 2003). Unfortunately, a recent systematic review (Wang et al 2008) found no statistically significant evidence for the effectiveness of reflexology, except in urinary problems associated with multiple sclerosis. Others are inconclusive, for example for constipation (Bishop et al 2003) and irritable bowel syndrome (Tovey et al 2002) and for stimulating ovulation (Holt et al 2008).

Within women's health, two trials have investigated the effects of reflexology on premenstrual syndrome, one early study showing a positive outcome (Oleson & Flocco 1993), whilst the other did not (Kim et al 2004). This is an interesting situation, because, as the methodology in complementary medicine research has improved – at least in the eyes of the medical profession – the number of studies with positive outcomes has declined. Very few investigations meet the "gold standard" of the randomised controlled trial (RCT), which has resulted in very negative feedback from authorities conducting systematic reviews of reflexology. Some systematic reviews of treatments for a particular condition include one or two studies on reflexology, but the therapy tends to fare poorly when compared to studies investigating the conventional management of particular conditions (Bamigboye & Smith 2007, Williamson et al 2002). It is no longer sufficient to promote only the relaxation effects of reflexology or the impact of touch on stress and pain. If reflexology is to be accepted as a clinical profession in its own right, there will need to be evidence of effectiveness, safety and the mechanism of action. Furthermore, these will need, where feasible, to be randomised, blinded and controlled trials, to comply with the criteria for acceptable research methodology.

One recent study (Mackereth et al 2009) compared the effects of reflexology and progressive muscle relaxation on people with multiple sclerosis, using a crossover design with a 4-week break between modalities and measuring salivary cortisol levels, heart rate, and systolic and diastolic blood pressure, as well as anxiety levels, before and after the weekly sessions. However, whilst most changes were statistically significant, the study was complicated at the crossover stage by the fact that the outcome measures did not return to the pre-treatment level in the 4-week break between one modality and the other, although there was a noticeable difference in anxiety levels in those who received reflexology. This study is important in that it begins to address some of the difficulties in terms of research methodology within reflexology and contributes to the emerging evidence base of the therapy and its evolution into a fully accepted profession.

Other contemporary investigations have considered the evidence for the mechanism of action. A study by Piquemal (2005) demonstrated a statistical correlation between five reflexology points on the feet (lung, liver, stomach, pancreas, and small intestine) and the dermatomes of the nervous system using an infra-cooled system connected to a computerised digital video card. The study appeared to show that reflexology acts by redistributing blood flow of the autonomic nervous system, presumably through a higher integrative nervous structure. Researchers at the Japanese Tohoku University School of Medicine elicited a direct correlation between certain reflexes in the feet and a response in the brain. A functional magnetic resonance imaging (fMRI) scan was used to observe responses in the brain when three specific reflex points on the feet were stimulated with a wooden stick – the reflex zones for the eye, the shoulder and the small intestine. The fMRI scans showed that the brain responded to stimulation of the feet, and also showed somatosensory areas for the eye, shoulder and small intestine (Nakamura et al 2008).

There are limited studies specifically dealing with pregnancy and childbirth. Mollart's single-blind study (2003) randomly assigned 55 women with gestational leg oedema to receive relaxation reflexology, reflexology treatment with specific lymphatic drainage techniques or rest, but found the results inconclusive, although the women reported most relief of discomfort with the specific reflexology treatment. Tipping and Mackereth (2000) focused on the establishment and maintenance of lactation with reflexology in mothers whose babies were in the Special Care Baby Unit, but attributed any apparent effects to a rebalancing of homeostasis, relaxation and relief of stress, which could be achieved with any touch or relaxation therapy. Similarly, Pourghaznein and Ghafari (2006) found a reduction in the severity of fatigue in pregnant women who received reflexology compared to a control group, but this too could merely have been the relaxation response from a manual therapy. McNeill et al (2006) explored the possible effects on the progress and outcome of labour in women who received reflexology towards the end of pregnancy compared to a group of women who did not, but showed no real statistical differences, apart from the use of inhalational analgesia.

CONCLUSION

Reflexology is a discrete complementary therapy profession in its own right with a developing body of knowledge to underpin practice. Whilst there is some way to go before it is accepted fully by the conventional medical professions, dedicated practitioners working at an advanced clinical level and those involved in academic work within higher education establishments are exploring the benefits, mechanism of action and physiological and psychological effects of reflexology in a variety of clinical specialties. The main emphasis of reflexology is on restoring and maintaining homeostasis, aiding relaxation and easing symptoms of stress.

RZT is a distinct sub-specialty of generic reflexology which has a tradition of direct application to and interaction with conventional healthcare and which is particularly relevant to maternity care. In addition to the relaxation factor, RZT can be used to treat or prevent exacerbation of many symptoms and pathological conditions, although of course it does not replace conventional medical management. Structural RZT is a contemporary variation of RZT which, in addition, focuses on deviations in the musculoskeletal system and the ways in which they may affect the body and mind. In maternity care, structural RZT can be particularly appropriate for easing aches and pains resulting from hormonal and weight-related physiology, as well as offering a new perspective on the aetiology of these complaints and a range of new techniques – or tools – with which to treat them.

Clinical practice of structural reflex zone therapy in maternity care

2

CHAPTER CONTENTS

AIMS OF STRUCTURAL REFLEX ZONE THERAPY IN PREGNANCY AND CHILDBIRTH

Reflexology and other complementary therapies have become extremely popular amongst pregnant women in recent years. Globally, there is considerable interest in the use of complementary therapies or natural remedies during pregnancy and childbirth, either through self-administration of substances available in health food stores or by consulting an independent practitioner (Hodgson et al 2007, Skouteris et al 2008). Some women may already have used complementary therapies prior to pregnancy, whereas others will wish to seek natural alternatives to drugs and medical interventions during the antenatal and intrapartum periods. In the UK, reflexology is classified by the House of Lords (2000) as being one of the Group 2 "supportive" therapies; in other words it is considered to be less well regulated and researched than the "top five" complementary therapies of Group 1. However, it appears, together with massage, aromatherapy, shiatsu (acupressure), hypnotherapy and others, to be amongst the most popular of the therapies generally available in the UK today. Acupuncture, osteopathy and chiropractic, herbal medicine and homeopathy are the other main therapies accessed by the general public, but these tend to be used for treatment of specific conditions, whereas the supportive therapies are frequently sought for relaxation on a regular basis. Indeed, the fast-paced life which women lead today indicates a real need for a means of "slowing down" and complementary therapies offer a range of choices to assist in this process.

Added to this is the parlous state of the UK maternity services, with public dissatisfaction exacerbated by adverse media coverage. Women embark on pregnancy with real fears about staff shortages, believing that they will have no maternity professional to whom they can turn during pregnancy or after birth and that they may be left unattended in labour. Many worry about the need for (sometimes unnecessary) tests and investigations and the chances of intervention in labour. In addition, these maternity-specific fears are compounded by reports of "superbugs", lack of resources and risks of medical errors in the contemporary National Health Service (NHS). For many, pregnancy is the first contact with the NHS but they may already have unrealistic expectations, which in themselves can contribute to increased fear, anxiety and tension.

Women who have left motherhood until perhaps their late thirties, as is now common, may have more disposable income than mothers-to-be had in previous decades and they are increasingly prepared to pay for services such as complementary therapies, which allow them that precious "me time" which can be so elusive to the working woman. Furthermore, reflex zone therapy (RZT) can be effective at relieving many of the physical symptoms of pregnancy – symptoms which pregnant women who are still working are less prepared to endure than their 20th century counterparts. In doing so, reflexology may also prevent physiological problems deteriorating into pathological complications, for example helping to maintain a relatively normal blood pressure and preventing the onset of more severe pre-eclampsia. In labour, reflexology provides a nurturing support to alleviate or reduce the mother's perception of contraction pain and assist in making her feel more comfortable. Reflex zone therapy goes one step further in offering an alternative means of dealing with some of the specific complications which may occur, for example accelerating labour which is failing to progress or assisting in placental separation when the third stage is prolonged. Postnatally, RZT can again help to reduce anxiety, aid recovery from birth, help with adaptation to parenthood and facilitate the establishment of breast feeding, and be used to treat minor complications following delivery, including pain and discomfort, retention of urine and inadequate milk supply.

Thus, reflexology offers a potential source of relief, both physiological and psychological. RZT should not, however, be interpreted as a replacement for orthodox midwifery and, where needed, medical care and practitioners must define their practice boundaries in the best interests of the mother and baby.

> **Box 2.1** Aims of structural reflex zone therapy in maternity care
>
> - To enhance maternal – and, indirectly, fetal – wellbeing during pregnancy through relaxation, by restoring and maintaining physical, psychological and emotional homeostatic balance
> - To provide the expectant mother with opportunities for time to herself for rest and relaxation, and with a "listening ear" to allow her to express her concerns
> - To complement normal midwifery/medical investigations by detecting, from a manual and visual examination of the feet, any existing or developing health issues which may impact on the progress and outcome of the pregnancy, labour and puerperium
> - To relieve symptoms and discomforts of pregnancy, labour and the postnatal period by promoting the mother's innate self-healing capacity and facilitating her coping mechanisms
> - To support the mother during labour and birth by aiding relaxation and reducing fear, pain and tension, which will contribute towards normal progress and outcomes
> - To prevent minor deviations from normal developing into medical/obstetric complications and to assist in reducing the severity of any complications which do arise

PROFESSIONAL ISSUES FOR MIDWIVES AND REFLEXOLOGISTS

RZT, as a clinical modality, requires the same degree of professional accountability as any other area of healthcare, both conventional and complementary. Practitioners should provide safe, effective treatments – which do no harm – in a professional manner, complying with all ethical and legal requirements and basing treatment on contemporary evidence-based theory and practice.

This is especially pertinent in maternity care because the National Institute for Health and Clinical Excellence (NICE), which produces guidelines for safe healthcare practice, has stated that there is "insufficient evidence" of the safety or effectiveness of complementary therapies in pregnancy and that, therefore, expectant mothers should be discouraged from using them (National Collaborating Centre 2008). Unfortunately this recommendation fails to take account of the fact that pregnant women are increasingly self-administering natural remedies and consulting complementary therapists and will continue to do so *despite* government advice to the contrary. It is also inaccurate, in that there is some evidence, albeit limited, for the effectiveness of reflexology and other touch therapies such as massage and aromatherapy, and an increasing number of small-scale studies in maternity complementary therapies (see Chapter 1). Furthermore, this lack of randomised controlled trials does not, of course, mean that reflexology has no place in maternity care, despite a need for more collation of any possible adverse effects and hazards. The implications for the practice of RZT within maternity care are, therefore, to work within currently accepted boundaries, basing treatments on contemporary theories of the therapy and relating this to individual physiology and care. This suggests an ultra-cautious approach, rather than a somewhat maverick evangelical attitude to the purported value of reflexology. Only by demonstrating to clients, and to colleagues with little or no understanding of reflexology, that women derive benefits which do not compromise materno-fetal health and wellbeing will this specialty evolve and become more integrated into conventional maternity care.

Education and training

Reflexologists wishing to specialise in treating pregnant and childbearing mothers should ensure they have adequate preparation, beyond their initial pre-registration training, to enable them to practise safely. It is essential that therapists have a thorough understanding of reproductive physiology and potential pathology (complications) during pregnancy, labour and the puerperium, an appreciation of the conventional maternity services and an awareness of their role and responsibilities when working with pregnant women. The core curriculum for reflexology now requires an introduction to working with maternity clients but does not prepare therapists, at the point of registration, to specialise in this area and considers pregnancy to be a subject best suited to specific continuing professional development including both theoretical study and supervised clinical practice (O'Hara 2006). Those with a qualification in generic reflexology also require additional preparation to treat women with specific conditions during pregnancy, labour and the puerperium, especially if they are not familiar with RZT techniques.

Conversely, midwives (and other conventional maternity care professionals such as health visitors) should be able to relate the principles of reflexology to obstetric theory, preferably through having completed a course specifically covering reflexology in maternity care. It is not acceptable to assume that a qualification in generic reflexology adequately equips them to treat pregnant mothers whilst working concomitantly as a midwife, especially in an institutional setting, and it may be necessary to undertake additional preparation to assist midwives to apply the principles of the therapy to the physiology of individual mothers. The Nursing and Midwifery Council (NMC) permits midwives (and nurses) to use complementary therapies such as reflexology in conjunction with their normal practice, on condition that they have adequate and appropriate training, can justify their actions and use all available theory and evidence to support their practice, in the best interests of the mother and baby (NMC 2008). In addition, midwives using RZT in their practice (or any other complementary therapies) have an obligation to maintain professional updating in both their midwifery and their RZT practice.

Legal issues

There are specific issues of accountability to consider when treating pregnant, labouring or newly delivered mothers. Legally, the only professionals who may take sole responsibility for the care of pregnant and childbearing women are midwives (the lead professional in the majority of births), doctors or midwifery/medical students under supervision, except in an emergency situation. This rule originates from the 1951 Midwives' Act and remains a requirement within the Nurses and Midwives Act 2001; it is designed to protect mothers and babies to ensure safe births. By inference, therefore, all therapies

Table 2.1 Educational requirements for maternity reflex zone therapy practice	
Pregnancy and childbirth	Reflexology
• Thorough understanding of reproductive anatomy and physiology • Pathology – impact of pregnancy on pre-existing medical conditions; complications of pregnancy, labour and the puerperium • Conventional maternity care services – antenatal care, investigations, personnel; labour and postnatal care • Role and responsibilities of the therapist when treating pregnant, labouring or newly delivered mothers in private practice and when integrated into the conventional maternity services • Relevant legal, ethical and professional issues • Dealing with emergencies	• Thorough working knowledge of reflex zone therapy (RZT) points • Understanding of mechanism of action of RZT • Indications, contraindications and precautions to RZT in general and to maternity care in particular • Effects, reactions, dangers and complications of RZT in general and in relation to pregnancy and childbirth in particular • Application of RZT to pregnancy and childbirth physiology and pathology • Awareness of potential interactions of RZT treatment with conventional maternity care, e.g. drugs

must be *complementary*, rather than alternative to conventional maternity care, and all practitioners should consider ways of developing communication links between local midwives/obstetricians and appropriately trained complementary practitioners.

Reflexologists who are not midwives will need to ensure that the pregnant women who attend for treatment are also booked for antenatal care with a midwife or doctor; whether under NHS care or privately. Unfortunately, there is a current trend for some women to opt for unassisted birth (sometimes called "freebirthing" in which they choose to give birth unattended by any maternity care professional). It is against the law for anyone who is not a midwife or doctor, including the partner, a friend, doula or complementary practitioner, to agree to assist these women without midwifery or medical support and to do so may result in prosecution. A simple means of determining whether the mother is booked for conventional maternity care is for the therapist to request to see the maternity records (notes) from the midwife or doctor, as all women in the UK carry their own maternity records for the duration of the pregnancy and until the end of the postnatal period. (Women in early pregnancy may not be given their notes until after their antenatal booking appointment, blood tests and ultrasound scans have been completed, at about 14–16 weeks' gestation.)

It is also important for therapists to recognise the boundaries and limitations of their expertise. Reflexologists are not permitted to prescribe treatment outside the limits of their practice and should refrain from offering their pregnant clients any information which may conflict with that given by the midwife, or which may not be adequately related to pregnancy in general or the individual mother's condition in particular. It is all too easy to have the desire to help clients but inadvertently to give advice which is either inaccurate or out of date. An example of this would be dietary information which is neither based on contemporary Department of Health guidelines on nutrition in pregnancy nor on recent research evidence. Indeed, reflexologists who are not trained nutritionists should be wary of offering any clients, whether pregnant or not, well-meaning advice which could be detrimental, either through error or omission of the full facts. Additionally, therapists should not undertake any specific techniques from reflexology or any other therapy unless they are adequately informed of its relevance to the individual mother and can justify their actions. An example would be the use of reflexology or acupressure points on the feet in an attempt to stimulate contractions without understanding how the labour is progressing and whether the health of mother and baby is satisfactory.

Similarly, midwives employed by the NHS or in a private maternity institution and who are also reflexologists need to have very clear parameters for practice. They should only use reflexology in their midwifery practice if permission has been granted by the employing authority; failure to do so may invalidate their right to vicarious liability insurance cover when providing midwifery care to women who also receive RZT (Tiran 2008). Conversely, when working as a reflexologist in private practice, they should not undertake any aspects of care which would normally be construed as the responsibility of the midwife, unless they have notified their Intention to Practise midwifery in the relevant geographical area.

Whilst it is not yet mandatory for all those who provide healthcare in any form to be in possession of personal professional indemnity insurance cover, it would be wise for all practitioners to have appropriate cover. The Royal College of Midwives will cover midwives' practice of complementary therapies when in employment such as the NHS, and are currently negotiating to extend this to midwives practising independently, although care during birth may not be included in this (RCM, personal communication 2008). Reflexologists should ensure that their insuring body covers them to treat pregnant women and they may also need additional insurance when attending women in labour (available from the Federation of Antenatal Educators, see References and resources section).

Guidelines for practice

Employed midwives who have been given permission to use reflexology to enhance their care of mothers should ensure that there are guidelines and/or policies for practice, to protect the mothers and babies as well as to protect their own professional integrity. Guidelines should ideally include a rationale for using RZT within midwifery, relating this to contemporary available evidence, together with the parameters for practice. The initial and ongoing training needs of midwives practising RZT should be outlined, as well as the professional requirements such as supervision, mentoring, continuing professional development requirements and accountability. A policy for a maternity unit should include the criteria for those approved to practise RZT, the indications, contraindications and precautions to treatment, i.e. criteria for eligibility of mothers to receive RZT (see Contraindications and precautions, below).

A decision should be made locally, and specified in the unit guidelines, regarding practice parameters when midwives use RZT in combination with conventional maternity care. For example, is treatment prescribed in a formulaic manner or is the individual midwife allowed to adapt treatment according to the needs of the individual mother? There are advantages and disadvantages to both of these approaches. A set routine, especially for relaxation reflexology, standardises treatment, which can be helpful in terms of reducing the amount of writing required when recording treatments in the notes of individual mothers, since a unit "formula" can be adopted. This also forms the basis for audit, may demonstrate the effectiveness of a particular treatment for a specific condition and could be particularly significant in the event of any legal action being brought against the maternity unit (see Chapters 4–6). Conversely, a more holistic approach, in which the midwife determines the precise treatment required by each individual mother, is more in keeping with the holistic philosophy of reflexology, and may contribute to satisfaction of both the mother and the midwife.

Some maternity units require independent therapists to sign a disclaimer form before treating the mothers within the maternity unit. The reflexologist may be asked to confirm that s/he has adequate personal professional indemnity insurance cover and understands that, in the event of a legal negligence case being brought against the Trust, s/he is not covered by the Trust's vicarious liability insurance which supports employees. S/he may also need to sign an agreement acknowledging that the midwife and/or obstetrician legally retains overall responsibility for the care of the mother and baby and that, if complications occur during the course of the labour, the therapist will defer to the midwife and, if necessary, modify or cease RZT. For therapists working in independent practice or intending to accompany women in labour within the conventional maternity services, it may also be wise to develop some standard strategies for certain aspects of maternity RZT. An example of this is the use of a common routine for a simple relaxation treatment (see Appendix 1). Independent therapists should also obtain evidence of having current Criminal Records Bureau (CRB) clearance.

An interesting point can be made here for midwives about doulas who accompany women during their labour. Increasing numbers of mothers are requesting the services of a doula to accompany them as an advocate and supporter during labour and some are trained to use complementary therapies as part of this work. However, there are many incidents known to this author where doulas have attempted to use complementary therapies including reflexology or aromatherapy without adequate training, commonly having gleaned a few "tips" from colleagues. Whilst a well-trained doula can be invaluable for the mother, it is of concern that some have no knowledge or understanding of either the therapy or its application to childbirth and are consequently putting mothers' and babies' lives at risk. Midwives, who have the legal responsibility for the care of the mother, should ensure that therapists and doulas wishing to use complementary therapy are appropriately educated and insured to do so.

Consent, confidentiality and record keeping

Obtaining informed consent from the mother to receive reflexology is essential. The mother's consent should be recorded in the notes, but verbal consent is usually sufficient and the mother does not need to sign a consent form. Obtaining consent requires the mother to be given an explanation of what the treatment is, how it is thought to work, what will happen during the treatment, responses she can expect to experience during and after the session, and what is expected of her in terms of being a partner in her care. It must be stressed, especially if she is seeking RZT for a specific condition, that while it can be generally relaxing, treatment is *not* simply a foot massage and may not be completely free of discomfort. She should be informed that it is expected that she will give feedback on any discomforts or tenderness she experiences during the session and that, unlike massage, receiving treatment with RZT is not a passive event.

Where reflexology is offered as part of conventional maternity care, it can be difficult to explain the therapy in terms that can be understood and some women may be very sceptical about the potential effects. Some mothers may have specific spiritual or religious views which influence their desire (or otherwise) to receive complementary therapies and these need to be taken into account. The mother also has the right to refuse treatment, a fact which can occasionally be overlooked by enthusiastic midwives keen to supplement conventional midwifery care with a therapy which appears to be relaxing, nurturing and something of a luxury in today's NHS.

Both midwives and therapists should ensure that the mother understands the nature of the treatment, the reason for offering it and the possible effects, including potential reactions to treatment. In some women suffering a particular condition, such as "morning sickness" or severe backache, a healing crisis may be more than they can cope with and they should have the opportunity to decline treatment for this reason too. Obviously, no guarantees for success of the treatment should be made.

Confidentiality is also paramount and may occasionally be inadvertently compromised by therapists in the excitement of treating a client who is progressing towards such a momentous and normally joyous life event.

Concise yet comprehensive record keeping is a legal requirement for any healthcare professional. Under the Congenital Disability (Civil Liability) Act (1976) all maternity case records are required to be kept for 25 years, since any claims for negligence resulting in birth-related injuries can be brought to court by the affected person during this time. Although this is not a legal requirement for those who do not have overall responsibility for the mother's and baby's care, reflexologists would be wise to retain for the full 25-year period the records of pregnant women whom they have treated. Surprisingly this issue does not appear to have been recognised by companies providing indemnity insurance cover to complementary practitioners, the usual maximum duration for retention of records being quoted as 7–10 years.

Notes should be as comprehensive as possible, with reflexology treatments recorded either in words or on a specific diagrammatic chart of the feet, or both. For midwives it may be simpler to record RZT treatments within the normal antenatal, labour or postnatal sections of the mother's handheld notes, using words which will be understood by conventional personnel involved in delivering care. Midwives should also be aware that RZT treatment in labour should be identified on the partogram and cardiotocograph printout as appropriate, both when the midwife is providing the treatment or if a mother is accompanied in labour by a reflexologist or by a doula who uses this (or any other) therapy. A note should be made when RZT commences and when it has been completed in order that fetal and uterine responses to treatment can be observed.

Independent therapists should not write in the NHS notes but should keep a separate set, possibly providing a copy for the mother to keep. Therapists not wishing to store notes for 25 years could approach the local Head of Midwifery Services and request the notes to be kept with the mother's record in the hospital archives. Therapists attending women in labour who are being cared for by midwives with no complementary therapy knowledge should communicate their intentions and treatments to the midwife responsible for the mother's overall care so that a record can be made in the notes. Midwives are required to maintain contemporaneous notes – writing up as they go along so that nothing is forgotten – and reflexologists would be wise to adhere to this practice too. It is very easy, particularly in the fast-changing and dynamic event of labour, to forget to record something at the time or be unable to recall it accurately if notes are recorded in retrospect.

PREPARATION FOR TREATING PREGNANT AND CHILD-BEARING WOMEN WITH STRUCTURAL REFLEX ZONE THERAPY

It is important to prepare adequately prior to treating any pregnant woman with RZT. This includes preparing the environment, the practitioner and the mother.

The environment

The room in which treatment is conducted should be warm, quiet and private. If treatment is being given within a clinic or ward setting, consideration should be given both to the peacefulness of the room for the mother receiving treatment, and to the impact on other women in the area. Whilst music can be pleasant during a treatment given purely for relaxation, it may not be appropriate when midwives are providing clinical RZT for treatment of specific problems, particularly if these are of an emotional nature. If music is to be used in the treatment area, careful choice should be made from the excellent selection of relaxation DVDs available, to avoid more well-known music which may have particular memories for some women. Relaxation music incorporating water or waves is best avoided when treating expectant mothers, who experience frequency of micturition as a normal symptom of pregnancy and for whom the sound of water can increase their urge to urinate. A discreet, *silent* clock is useful to help time-keeping when mothers are being treated in a clinic setting.

There should be adequate ventilation, with windows which open in case the mother reacts to treatment and begins to feel hot, but a large towel or blanket should also be to hand as some women respond by shivering and feeling cold. Good lighting is *essential* to the inspection stage of the treatment process and the dim lighting beloved by so many therapists is to be actively discouraged unless treatment is given purely for relaxation. In this case it would be acceptable, after the inspection stage, to dim the lighting to a level at which the feet and the mother's facial and other reactions can still be observed.

Natural light is preferable, but if electric light is necessary, this should not shine directly into the mother's face, nor should it be behind the practitioner, as this will prevent the mother from seeing his/her face properly.

A small step or stool, strategically and safely placed to enable the mother to get onto the couch may be necessary if the couch does not have the facility to be raised or lowered. The mother should be discouraged from climbing onto the couch in such a way that her legs are widely abducted as this may cause or exacerbate any existing symphysis pubis discomfort. The couch should also have a back rest to enable her to sit up or the therapist should provide several pillows for support. Pregnant women should *never* be treated in the fully recumbent position, since this risks supine hypotension. It also prevents the dynamic two-way interaction necessary between the mother and practitioner. In RZT the client is not merely a passive recipient but is an active participant in the treatment process, at least at the commencement of the session when her answers to questions and reports of reactions to the treatment are required. A towel may be used on the couch to cover one of the mother's feet whilst working on the other, and padding beneath the knees can aid the mother's comfort, but care must be taken not to occlude circulation in the calves as this may increase the risk of deep vein thrombosis or cause added pressure on already uncomfortable varicosities. Padded wedges can be useful but the feet should be easily accessible and should not hang over the edge of the wedge or the end of the couch or bed. Conversely, if the mother is not very tall she may need to be positioned carefully so that her feet are at the end of the couch whilst remaining comfortably supported, yet enabling the therapist to reach her feet comfortably. If a fold-up lounger-style chair is used, as has recently become very popular for reflexology, it is acceptable for the mother to be in a slightly more reclining position, as the fabric of the chair is soft. This will not then cause the compression which leads to the supine hypotension of pregnancy, in which the inferior vena cava occludes blood flow returning to the heart, causing dizziness and a temporary reduction in oxygen supply to the fetus.

The chair or stool on which the practitioner sits should enable him/her to be comfortable, with his/her feet firmly on the floor. It should preferably have no side arms, as this will prevent adequate manoeuvring of the practitioner's arms during treatment. A possible alternative, when no couch is available, might be for the mother to sit in a comfortable reclining chair and for the therapist to sit on a small stool, lower than the mother's knees, with a pillow on her knees for the mother to rest her feet. This is more comfortable for the mother than having her feet up at the same level as the practitioner's knees, as would occur if both sat on a chair of equal height – this causes discomfort after a while in the popliteal space behind the knees. If a mother is to be treated whilst sitting or lying on her bed, either at home or in the hospital, the practitioner should give due consideration to his/her own posture. In the hospital it is usually possible to detach the end of the bed so that the therapist can sit at the end. At home this will probably not be possible and it would be inappropriate to sit on one side of the bed to reach the mother's feet, as this will cause discomfort for the therapist (and is not particularly professional or hygienic).

It is useful to have a glass of water, tissues and a vomit bowl nearby, as physiological or emotional reactions occur in some women, such as bursting into tears, feeling nauseated or starting to experience a "dripping" nose or sneezing. Midwives should have available the normal accoutrements of their practice, including a sphygmomanometer and stethoscope, Pinard's stethoscope or portable fetal heart monitor, as well as access to the mother's maternity notes. However, therapists who are not midwives should acknowledge the parameters of their personal practice and be wary of over-stepping these boundaries. Only therapists who have been trained to use medical tools correctly and interpret the results, so that they know when to act on those results, should have these in their treatment room.

In RZT *no* creams, lotions or powders are used as these can interfere with the ability to assess the feet fully or to grip them adequately to perform the treatment, although practitioners who have the relevant skills may choose to complete the relaxation component of treatment with a foot massage using base oils, with or without essential oils. If this is intended the oil massage of the feet should be performed *after* the reflexology treatment. However, it is not normal practice to combine different complementary therapies unless the practitioner is very experienced in using therapies specifically applied to pregnant women, as it is necessary to be able to recognise reactions to individual therapies and to differentiate these from the physiopathological symptoms of pregnancy. The use of essential oils in a vaporiser or the burning of incense sticks is *completely inappropriate* in a clinical setting, not least because not all women may like the aromas, but also because inhalation of the chemicals within the oils may be detrimental to the mother's health or interfere with her response to RZT.

The practitioner

The midwife or therapist must be in good health and should decline to treat a woman if s/he is feeling unwell or overtired. Midwives, in particular, should ensure they have adequate time away from their normal commitments to undertake RZT treatment, preferably (but perhaps somewhat unrealistically!) having had a short rest before beginning. Both the mother and the practitioner should make sure they have emptied their bladders; the midwife providing treatment should also ensure s/he is well hydrated and, if necessary, should have a drink of water before commencing treatment. If time allows s/he should eat a snack so that s/he is better able to cope with the energy transfer which can occur between client and therapist. The midwife must allow sufficient time to complete the session in an unhurried manner; this may require some re-allocation of other aspects of his/her work, or asking a colleague to cover for him/her. In the delivery suite or a ward setting it is especially important to hand over his/her bleep and the departmental drug keys to a colleague so that s/he will not be disturbed, and the use of a discreet sign on the door indicating that therapy is in progress should prevent unnecessary intrusions from others.

The practitioner should remove his/her watch and any jewellery such as rings and bracelets, in order to avoid scratching the mother. The mother should also be asked to remove her watch; this is for more esoteric reasons – reflexology involves an energy transfer and there should be no risk of interfering with the theoretical energy fields by being in contact with the magnetism of watches. A small container should be provided for the mother's jewellery and watch; she should not be permitted to rest the watch on her body during treatment as this will defeat the object. Similarly any toe rings should be removed as these may become uncomfortable during treatment, as well as interfering with the visual and manual examination.

The mother

Before undertaking treatment it is necessary to determine if the mother can receive RZT and to decide the nature of the treatment. When the mother telephones to arrange an appointment, it may be helpful to ask some pertinent questions, based on the absolute contraindications, to ensure that she is eligible for treatment (see Box 2.2). She should be asked *not* to wash her feet or use moist cleansing wipes to remove sweat and odour before attending for treatment, nor should she apply creams or lotions to the skin as this can interfere with the essential assessment of the feet, as well as the grip sequence. During this telephone conversation the mother can also be advised that it is preferable if small children do not accompany her, if at all possible, as this can detract from the overall benefits she may derive from treatment. However, if the mother is to be treated by the midwife in a clinic setting for a specific condition, this is not always practicable.

At the first appointment, a full medical, social and obstetric history should be carried out, or, if RZT is to be given by the midwife, the mother's handheld notes should be read for any relevant contraindications, precautions or pertinent issues. If treatment is to be given by an independent therapist, it is wise to ask the mother to bring her maternity notes with her. Even though the therapist may not be able to interpret all the terminology, the presence of the notes will assure him/her that the mother is booked for conventional maternity care, either via the National Health Service or privately. The

---

Box 2.2 Suggested items for discussion with the mother when booking her first appointment

- Gestation of pregnancy and general wellbeing to date
- Presenting problem/complaint (reason for treatment)
- Pre-existing major medical conditions, e.g. epilepsy, cardiac disorder, thyroid disease, diabetes, which may preclude her from receiving RZT
- Deep vein thrombosis or pulmonary embolism
- Diabetes mellitus – insulin-dependent or not
- Obstetric problems – multiple pregnancy, hypertension, vaginal bleeding
- Any recent hospital admission since becoming pregnant – and reason
- History of renal calculi or gallstones, presence of retained intrauterine contraceptive device
- Enquire whether she has informed her midwife if consulting independent therapist
- Advise her to bring her conventional maternity care (hand-held) notes with her
- Request that she does not wash or wipe her feet, nor apply creams/lotions
- Request that children are left with someone else if at all possible
- Ask her to let you know if she feels too unwell to attend for treatment

therapist should not write in the normal maternity notes (although it is acceptable to include a copy of his/her own record in the back of the notes) and should undertake his/her own assessment of the mother, based on the usual full history.

It is particularly relevant to be aware of any major medical or obstetric issues that may have a bearing on whether or not treatment is appropriate. This includes identifying a history of epilepsy, diabetes mellitus, hypertension, cardiac, cardiovascular, thyroid, renal, hepatic or psychiatric illness, as well as obtaining an account of any infertility, previous pregnancies, including any complications, miscarriages and terminations, labours and deliveries, and the current health of any children. Enquiries should be made about the progress of the current pregnancy: the gestation and number of fetuses, any vaginal bleeding, placental location (recorded on the ultrasound scan report in the notes), hypertension, threatened preterm labour and, as term approaches, the position and approximate size of the fetus.

A musculoskeletal history should be taken when the practitioner intends to use the structural RZT approach. This includes recording any previous fractures or other injuries or surgical procedures which may have a bearing on the aetiology or management of specific conditions. Asking the mother if she has ever been in a road traffic accident, a skiing or riding accident, or has ever had a fall down the stairs or from a bike, even when much younger, can give an indication of possible musculoskeletal misalignment. Any dental surgery should also be noted as difficult extractions, bridges, caps, crowns or other structural dental work may impact on the position and function of the head, jaw, mouth and neck (see Chapter 1). Occasionally it is useful to enquire whether or not the mother knows the type of birth she had, i.e. the type of delivery her mother experienced, as a difficult delivery may have affected musculoskeletal alignment, which, in some cases, is lifelong. When asking about the obstetric history it is also useful to focus on any backache, sciatica, symphysis pubis discomfort, carpal tunnel syndrome, or similar problems experienced in previous pregnancies, as well as any history of breech presentation or fetal malposition, since these may recur, especially if they are related to misalignment (see Chapters 4 and 5). It is also useful to undertake a physical assessment of pelvic symmetry which may give an indication of any generalised musculoskeletal misalignment. This simple technique involves the mother standing, with no shoes on, facing the practitioner, who places the thumbs of his/her two hands on the iliac crests (anterior hip bones) and rests the fingers of each hand on the back of the pelvis. S/he then asks the mother to step carefully away from him/her, while the practitioner keeps his/her thumbs stationary. Although this is not a precise assessment, if the level of the practitioner's two thumbs are seen to be at different levels this may indicate that one of the mother's hips is higher than the other, giving the suggestion of overall musculoskeletal misalignment.

If the mother presents for RZT because of a specific condition or physiological discomfort such as backache or constipation, a history of the current complaint should also be recorded, together with any other relevant information. It is also necessary to determine the cause of the problem by considering the differential diagnosis. For example, in the event of backache, the practitioner may focus particularly on the musculoskeletal history, ergonomics and postural habituation, but should ensure that the cause is not due to other problems such as urinary tract infection, severe constipation or even the onset of labour. The mother's psychological and emotional state should also be assessed, including the way in which she responds to the complaint and how she is coping with it. It may be useful, for example, to use a simple Likert scale measurement to obtain a perception of the degree to which the mother is suffering; a comparison can then be made after and between treatments to identify if the mother feels any improvement in her overall wellbeing. For example, the mother may present with nausea, vomiting, heartburn and constipation in early pregnancy and self-assess the severity of her symptoms as 10/10 (or even more!). After RZT, the heartburn may have subsided, constipation may have improved and perhaps the number of vomiting occasions has reduced. Using the same measurement scale, the mother will hopefully recognise that, even though nausea persists and she is still occasionally sick, she feels generally better than before she received treatment, RZT having perhaps enhanced her coping abilities.

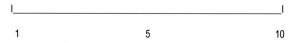

1	5	10

Ask the mother to grade, on a scale on 1–10, her subjective assessment of the severity of her symptoms, both before and after reflex zone treatment. This will help her to recognise the extent to which she feels better.

Fig. 2.1 Simple scale to assess severity of symptoms

It is also necessary to assess the mother before each treatment, as her condition may change between appointments. The therapist or midwife should enquire about the current state of maternal and fetal wellbeing: her bowels, micturition, vaginal discharge, development of any new symptoms such as headaches, visual disturbances or excessive oedema, which can be a sign of worsening pre-eclampsia, and fetal movements. An evaluation of the mother's response to the previous treatment should also be made, which may give an indication of success and whether the treatment needs to be adapted for this appointment. This should include responses to treatment in the first 24 hours after the session and in the period since then until the current appointment. If there is any doubt about the condition of either the mother or fetus treatment should be cancelled or postponed until medical or midwifery advice has been sought and it has been deemed acceptable for the mother to continue to receive RZT.

Once the history has been taken, a decision has been made about the treatment and the mother has given her consent, she should be asked if she wishes to empty her bladder and to turn her mobile telephone to silent mode. If she has small children with her, some means of keeping them occupied for at least 25–30 minutes should be sought. The mother should then be assisted into a position ready for the visual examination, if RZT is being given during pregnancy or after delivery (in labour, this element is usually omitted).

RZT is a powerful clinical tool and, as such, must be used with respect. Although RZT is a natural therapy, it is not without some risk and practitioners should be aware of these before commencing any treatment. It is particularly important to recognise the contraindications and precautions in order to identify which pregnant women should not have treatment or whose session should be modified as a result of the mother's specific condition. RZT is not contraindicated in pregnancy; indeed, it may be an extremely valuable aid to wellbeing and health. However, there are some women who will be unsuited to receive RZT during their pregnancies, either for general medical reasons or for specific obstetric indications, and it is necessary to identify these mothers prior to booking an appointment, to avoid a wasted journey and unfulfilled expectation of treatment (see Box 2.2). It has been stressed already that RZT is a clinical modality, which in the case of pregnant and childbearing women, should always be combined with conventional maternity care. An ultra-cautious approach will gain more credibility and acceptance from medical and midwifery colleagues and will be safer for mothers and their babies, than attempting to stretch the boundaries too quickly and too far.

Any therapy, performed inappropriately, may pose risks to the mother and/or baby. The practitioner has a responsibility to work within her personal level of understanding and her ability to apply generic principles to pregnancy-specific conditions. It is important to recognise when the woman's condition warrants more specialised treatment, and when it is appropriate to refer back for conventional medical management. Reflexologists must be able to differentiate between women whose condition is merely physiological and those with impending or actual pathological complications, either general illnesses, such as influenza, or obstetric problems, for example fulminating pre-eclampsia. Most importantly, any intuitive feeling on the part of the practitioner that RZT could compromise the maternal or fetal condition is an indication that treatment should not be performed until the individual circumstances change.

First trimester treatment

In many traditional reflexology textbooks, pregnancy, especially the first trimester, is classified as a contraindication to treatment, but this appears to be more a protection for the therapist than based on any real evidence that treatment at this time is "dangerous". Many reflexologists seem to feel that their treatment will cause miscarriage, but of course this is not true if it is performed safely and appropriately. Miscarriage is a response of the mother's body to a pregnancy which is not meant to be. However, treatment during the first trimester should *always* be undertaken with care, preferably performed only by very experienced therapists with a comprehensive knowledge of relevant physio-pathology. On the other hand, some women may have been receiving reflexology for an unrelated condition, or simply for relaxation, before they become aware of the pregnancy; others may choose not to inform anyone in the early weeks, in the superstitious belief that it may jeopardise the pregnancy. Therefore, *all* women of reproductive age who attend for RZT should be asked about their menstrual cycle: if they are unable to recall the date of their last period, if they think they may be pregnant or if they are actively trying to conceive, they should be treated *as if* they are pregnant, with the attendant precautions.

Women with a history of previous miscarriage need to be treated very cautiously. They may desire the relaxation effect of a manual therapy, as they will feel very anxious, but it may be wise only to perform simple foot massage and reflexology relaxation movements, as opposed to specific RZT techniques, until they have exceeded the gestation at which previous miscarriages occurred. Also, as the causes of, and predisposing factors to spontaneous abortion are multifactorial, reflexology should not be viewed as a preventative treatment against miscarriage. Unless it is confirmed that stress is the only factor, treatment should not be given in a misguided attempt to deal with the causes. Women with a more complicated medical or obstetric history, including those with an *in situ* suture to control cervical incompetence, should not be treated in pregnancy. If the therapist decides that specific reflex zone techniques are not appropriate and substitutes a gentle foot massage, the use of base oils is permissible, but no essential oils should be used to avoid the risk of any pharmacological adverse effects. Care should be taken not to massage the heels too briskly, as the heels are the reflex zones for the pelvic organs. Although there is no evidence that this brisk massage can over-stimulate the pelvic area, neither is there evidence to the contrary, and it would not be possible categorically to deny that, in the event of a miscarriage occurring, it was not as a consequence of the therapy.

Infertility

A word here about infertility: There is a common theory amongst the general public who use reflexology that it can "treat" infertility, but this of course is not entirely true. As with miscarriage, infertility (or more correctly, subfertility) also has a very complex – and often inter-related – aetiology and it may be impossible to help some women to conceive, either with conventional medicine or with complementary therapies.

Infertility is not, in itself, an absolute contraindication to RZT, but, once a woman has committed herself to investigations and conventional infertility treatment under the care of a specialist infertility gynaecologist, it should be performed with care and only after communication with the doctor. The woman may benefit from the relaxation effect whilst awaiting her first appointment, and during the period of time in which the various uncomfortable and embarrassing investigations are undertaken. If assisted reproduction, such as in vitro fertilisation (IVF), is offered, no reflexology should be performed whilst the woman is taking drugs to aid ovulation, either by nasal spray, oral drugs or skin patches. The released oocytes are then retrieved surgically and fertilisation takes place in the laboratory – during this worrying time of waiting reflexology can be very helpful in keeping the woman calm. However, once the fertilised blastocyst is re-implanted into the woman's uterus, reflexology should again be withheld until either pregnancy has been confirmed and has become established (i.e. the end of the first trimester) or menstruation has occurred because conception has failed (see also Chapter 4).

Women with medical conditions

Certain medical conditions are not consistent with RZT treatment, particularly during pregnancy, as pre-existing conditions often worsen at this time, or may adversely affect the prognosis or progress of the pregnancy. In many cases, where a woman has been taking medication for her condition this may need to be changed for the duration of the pregnancy and this, in itself, can upset the stability of the condition, quite apart from the effect on pregnancy physiology.

There are some medical conditions which are absolute contraindications to RZT, especially during pregnancy. Women with epilepsy *should never be treated with RZT*; epilepsy can become very unstable in the presence of pregnancy hormones and women will be under the care of both the obstetrician and a physician. Also, in some women, the relaxation effect from the treatment can be sufficient to trigger a fit; so therapists who choose to treat epileptic women – and who feel they can justify their actions – should be competent and confident to deal with a fit, if one should occur.

Cardiac conditions are also an absolute contraindication, unless they are exceptionally minor. Most cardiac pathology usually worsens by at least one degree in pregnancy because of the impact of the increased blood supply, fluctuations in blood pressure and hypertrophy of the heart in an already compromised cardiovascular system.

Other conditions present problems which suggest that RZT should be used cautiously, rather than being completely contraindicated. Thyroid function is exacerbated in pregnancy; therefore, mothers with an overactive thyroid need to be treated carefully to avoid inadvertent additional stimulation of the thyroid gland via the corresponding reflex zone. Whilst it may be assumed that an underactive thyroid gland could be stimulated with RZT, women with hypothyroidism on medication should also be treated cautiously, in order to prevent exacerbation of the pharmacological actions of the drugs.

Diabetic mothers should be assessed individually prior to each treatment. Those with pre-existing or gestational (pregnancy-induced) diabetes who do not require insulin (diet-controlled) may be treated with care, but may best be advised to eat a small carbohydrate meal beforehand to avoid hypoglycaemia occurring as a result of inadvertent over-stimulation of the reflex zone for the pancreas. Mothers who are insulin-dependent, whose pregnancies and fetal wellbeing may be compromised by their medical condition, should not normally receive RZT, unless it is performed with good justification by a midwife who is an experienced reflexologist.

RZT is known to lower blood pressure (Ejindu 2007, Lee 2006) and may compound the effects of anti-hypertensive drugs. In addition, pregnant women, notably those in the second trimester, often have a below-baseline blood pressure due to the vasodilatory effects of progesterone. It is for this reason that pregnant women should never be treated in a totally recumbent position, and care should be taken at the end of any treatment (even when the mother is sitting upright) to ensure that she arises from the couch slowly, with support, to prevent postural hypotension. Fainting can be both a response to treatment and a physiological effect of pregnancy and it is necessary to identify the causative factor in the event of the woman feeling faint.

Clinical practice of structural reflex zone therapy in maternity care

It is often stated that carcinoma is a contraindication to complementary therapy, but this is not absolute. Cancer patients frequently obtain great comfort from light reflexology treatments of short duration, performed by therapists who understand the pathology and medical treatment effects of the individual's condition (Quattrin et al 2006). However, in pregnancy, extra care needs to be taken and the novice would be best advised to refrain from giving any specific treatment unless under the direction of an appropriately qualified midwife with RZT experience. Realistically, it is unlikely that therapists in private practice will come into contact with women who are both pregnant and living with cancer, although occasionally midwives may be presented with pregnant clients with existing or previous breast or cervical cancer or those who have received suspect results from routine investigations. These women may be given light reflexology treatments for relaxation but no stimulating or sedating techniques should be employed.

Women with systemic infections and/or pyrexia should not be treated, as RZT has a warming effect which may exacerbate the signs and symptoms, and the mother may feel too unwell to benefit from treatment. Although the physiological temperature rises by 1°C in pregnancy, antenatal pyrexia is always abnormal and may herald the onset of an acute infection, which may have an adverse effect on the materno–fetal unit. For example, a urinary tract infection, which is not uncommon in pregnancy, may lead to severe pyelonephritis or to preterm labour in susceptible women if left untreated. Furthermore, the therapist may be at risk of contracting the mother's infection, or negative energy may be transmitted from the mother to the therapist causing him/her to feel tired and lethargic.

On the other hand, whilst infections and lesions on the feet, such as verrucae and corns, can be unpleasant, these are not definite contraindications to treatment and can actually be relevant as an aid to diagnosis during visual examination of the feet. It is the prerogative of the individual practitioner to decide whether or not she wishes to treat women who have any of these conditions. Some authorities suggest that the therapist could wear thin disposable gloves, but this interferes with the sensitivity of the practitioner to detect variations in the feet, and detracts from the human contact aspect of the treatment. It is not, therefore, realistically a viable option as a general rule, but may be helpful in cases where there is acute eczema or mycosis of the feet (athlete's foot). Women with more serious foot-related problems, such as a fracture or amputation, may not be able to receive RZT on that foot, but could be treated on the other foot using the zone concept or on their hands (although if carpal tunnel syndrome is present this may be uncomfortable and treatment may be less effective as it will not be as easy to apply pressure). Similarly, it may be uncomfortable for women with varicose veins to receive treatment on their feet, but the hands may be a suitable alternative.

Women who have a history of pulmonary embolism at any time should not be treated using RZT, as the risks of further embolic episodes during pregnancy are high and these women will be under strict medical supervision and usually taking anticoagulant drugs. Any woman currently taking anticoagulant medication such as warfarin or similar drugs should not be treated. Those with a history of deep vein thrombosis (DVT) in the 6 months prior to pregnancy, or during a previous pregnancy should be treated with extreme caution, and attention should be given to careful positioning of the legs on the chair, avoiding occlusion of circulation in the calves. If there is any redness, inflammation or pain in either calf, which may indicate thrombo-embolic disorder, treatment should be discontinued until DVT has been excluded. This applies also to the postnatal period when the clotting mechanism of the blood has changed to accommodate blood loss in labour and there is then a temporarily increased risk of thrombosis. In mothers with varicose veins, manual palpation should not be performed directly over the varicosed area and if the localised skin is inflamed or broken down, a wider area should be avoided. In women who have inflammation of the lymphatic system, either generalised, or localised in the legs and feet, such as behind the knees or in the groin, RZT is contraindicated as the increased lymphatic and venous return occurring during treatment may overload an already compromised system. Gentle treatment may be performed on mothers with oedema if the skin is not too tense and painful, and can be helpful in reducing swelling (Mollart 2003). Women with arthritic disease involving the feet should not be treated during an active phase.

It is generally considered that RZT should not be performed immediately post-operatively since the individual may feel too unwell and there is a risk that any post-operative complications may be masked by responses to treatment, or vice versa. However, mothers who have had a Caesarean section or manual removal of placenta, but who are otherwise fit and healthy, can receive relaxation RZT and short treatments for specific problems, such as retention of urine, once they have recovered from the immediate effects of the anaesthetic, usually after 24 hours. Women who require surgery during pregnancy should not be treated until well past the post-operative phase, as any surgery, whether obstetric or for incidental medical conditions (e.g. appendicitis) can interfere with the stability of the pregnancy.

"Foreign bodies"

From experience, RZT seems to be particularly effective at "moving things along tubes", including faeces along the intestines or ear wax along the Eustachian tube. However, this means that it also has the potential, in unskilled hands, to move foreign bodies out of place, including gallstones, renal calculi or heart pacemakers, although it is highly unlikely that pregnant women will have a pacemaker *in situ*. However, mothers with a history of calculi in the gall bladder or kidney should be treated very cautiously, or not at all, as it is theoretically possible to move a stone from a duct where it is situated relatively undisturbed, into a smaller duct which would significantly increase pain. Conversely, of course, it could be argued that reflexology could facilitate expulsion of a stone, but it would be inappropriate to treat a pregnant woman with this condition as any pain or complication could affect the maintenance and progress of the pregnancy.

Of more relevance to treating young women of reproductive years (prior to conception) is the very real possibility of displacing an intrauterine contraceptive device (IUCD), leading to pain and discomfort at the very least and an unanticipated risk of unwanted pregnancy. A case is known to this author of a woman whose coil became dislodged within 8 hours of RZT treatment (not performed by the author!). It is perhaps this principle which also leads inexperienced therapists to believe that RZT can displace the "foreign body" which is the embryo in early pregnancy, but this would only be the case in an unstable pregnancy. However, occasionally a woman will become pregnant whilst a contraceptive coil is in the uterus; it is imperative that *no* work on the reflex zone for the uterus is undertaken at any time during pregnancy.

Marquardt advises that patients with major psychiatric disorders should only be treated under medical supervision and by experienced therapists who can assess the current state of the psychosis or other conditions such as schizophrenia (Marquardt 1983:29). The rationale given for this is that any medication may mask the normal responses to RZT. In pregnancy, psychological disorders can worsen because of the hormonal upheaval and it may be difficult to identify whether behavioural or emotional changes are the result of a pathological exacerbation of the condition, a therapy-induced reaction or some other factor. The relaxation effect alone may be insufficient indication for performing RZT.

Similarly, care should be taken when treating women with addictive behaviours, such as drug or alcohol dependency. The physiological impact of treatment may potentiate the actions of any drugs, both those used recreationally and those given therapeutically, whilst the relaxation effects of treatment may inadvertently indulge the woman's addictive personality. Furthermore, the requirement of mothers to work in partnership with the therapist for optimum wellbeing may be compromised by women who do not feel committed to making lifestyle changes. As a general rule, it may be best to treat these women with RZT only for specific physical conditions rather than with an ongoing course of treatment for relaxation. Conversely, where therapy is provided within a psychiatric environment in conjunction with medical management, midwifery care and social interventions, RZT can be a valuable aid to recovery.

Obstetric contraindications and precautions

Pregnancy is a time of huge physiological and psychological disruption and this must be taken into account when deciding whether it is appropriate to treat an expectant mother. We have already discussed issues pertaining to the pre-conception period and the first trimester, but after about 14 weeks' gestation, many women will enjoy and benefit from RZT throughout their pregnancy. An assessment should be made at each appointment to ensure that the mother and fetal wellbeing remains stable, and if any changes occur which are beyond the normal parameters of gestational adaptation, treatment may need to be postponed or adapted.

Some obstetric complications signify that RZT is not appropriate. *Any* vaginal bleeding is abnormal in pregnancy. In the first trimester this may be a threatened miscarriage and no treatment should be performed until bleeding has subsided and the pregnancy has progressed to a stage where is appears stable. In later pregnancy, bleeding from the vagina is usually placental in origin, either from a normally situated placenta, in which a small area becomes detached from the uterine wall (placental abruption), or from a low-lying placenta (placenta praevia). Until the cause of the bleeding is known no treatment should be undertaken. Women with a known grade 3 or 4 placenta praevia should not be treated *at all* during their pregnancy. Those with a grade 1 or 2 placenta praevia may be able to receive care near term, once it has been shown by ultrasound scan that the lower uterine segment has stretched sufficiently for the edge of the placenta to be out of reach of the cervical os. However, any direct stimulation or sedation of the reflex points for the uterus is to be totally avoided. If, after delivery, a mother has suffered a postpartum haemorrhage, she may be anaemic, tired and unwell; RZT is not appropriate at this early stage, although simple relaxation treatment can be given after the immediate recovery period.

If a mother experiences abdominal pain that is shown to have a pathological cause rather than merely being due to stretching of the abdominal musculature, RZT should be withheld until a diagnosis has been made, and a decision can then be taken about pursuing the course of treatment. Mothers with strong Braxton Hicks contractions in the third trimester should be treated with care, although sometimes RZT can be a valuable aid to easing the discomfort. If there is any risk or sign of preterm labour, no treatment should be given until 37 weeks' gestation. This also applies to premature rupture of the membranes. Grande multiparae are more at risk of preterm labour and should, therefore, be treated extremely gently prior to term and only by midwives experienced in using RZT.

Women with multiple pregnancies suffer many symptoms related to their increased weight and hormonal effects, and may benefit from RZT. However, whilst the pregnancy may be "normal" for a multiple pregnancy, with no apparent complications, it is not a pregnancy without risk, and RZT should be given cautiously. It is usually acceptable to treat a mother with an uncomplicated twin pregnancy but any woman expecting triplets or quadruplets should only be treated by very experienced midwife-reflexologists and it may be wise to offer only a simple relaxation treatment. Practitioners in independent practice *must* obtain midwifery or medical approval to proceed if the client has a twin pregnancy and should liaise regularly with the conventional maternity care team. Independent reflexologists should not treat mothers carrying more than two babies.

Blood pressure fluctuates physiologically and between individuals in pregnancy. Therapists should understand these variations and be alert to any indications of pre-eclampsia. RZT is not contraindicated in the presence of mild pre-eclampsia but it is necessary to identify if this is becoming more serious; for example, the emergence of signs such as excessive oedema, or reports of symptoms such as headaches, nausea, right-sided abdominal pain and visual disturbances, which can signify internal oedema around major organs. In these cases treatment should be withheld and a medical opinion sought urgently. Mothers with mild pre-eclampsia who remain as out-patients may benefit from RZT, but once admitted for medical treatment for fulminating pre-eclampsia, RZT should be withheld. In the event of a previous history of eclampsia, RZT is contraindicated, since, despite the hypotensive effects of treatment, her condition may once again be very unstable and she will be under the close scrutiny of the obstetricians.

It must be remembered that, during pregnancy, the materno–fetal unit is a single entity and, therefore, consideration must be given to the effects on the baby. Often there is a noticeable change in the pattern of fetal movements during RZT, indicating a response by the fetus to the alterations in the mother's condition. Therefore, when fetal wellbeing is compromised by poor growth or a diagnosed abnormality, it may be wise not to treat the mother. Conversely, it could be reasoned that the increase in circulation thought to occur during treatment is productive, facilitating better transfusion of blood to the fetus. The decision whether or not to proceed with RZT will need to be based on the precise condition of the individual mother and fetus.

In labour, RZT can be undertaken by midwives caring for women, or by appropriately trained, insured and approved therapists, under the supervision of the midwife responsible for the mother's care (see Professional issues, above). However, it is essential that the practitioner is aware of the nature of the mother's progress, the efficacy of uterine contractions, descent of the fetal presenting part and adequacy of the bony pelvis, particularly prior to instigating any treatment designed to expedite delivery. It is *completely inappropriate* and ethically questionable for therapists to attempt to induce labour before the estimated delivery date, although specific techniques can be employed after this time, under the direction of the midwife, if this is not the therapist (see Chapter 5).

Short, intermittent treatments may be necessary during the first stage of labour rather than a single complete session, and they may need to be adapted according to the mother's contractions. The therapist may also need to be flexible (quite literally!) in order to give RZT if the mother has chosen to labour in a position other than sitting or lying semi-recumbent on the bed, for example, on "all fours" or over a birthing ball. RZT, like other manual therapies, can make the difference between a mother requiring pharmacological analgesia and managing to cope with the pain herself (Chang et al 2002, Feder et al 1994). However, RZT should be used with extreme caution if a mother decides to have intramuscular pethidine or another opioid analgesic, to prevent masking or exacerbation of reactions to either the drug or the treatment. Furthermore, the physiological responses to RZT may be affected more significantly in the presence of regional analgesia, such as epidural. Indeed, Lett (2000:227) states that:

> Medication alters the internal milieu, and the responses to RZT after … being given drugs may be faster or slower than usual. This also happens when there is sensory deprivation of any kind. For this reason it is inadvisable to use RZT at the same time as epidural anaesthesia. A very fine judgement is needed when treating those who are heavily medicated.

Although this author concurs with Lett's reasoning, experience suggests that careful RZT by the attending midwife is acceptable as a means of maintaining relaxation and calm for a mother whose labour may be beginning to deviate from normal. However, the parameters for practice in individual maternity units may preclude women with epidural analgesia in situ from receiving complementary therapies. In units where there is a low-risk, midwife-led birthing centre, mothers requiring epidural analgesia may be required to transfer to the high-risk delivery suite and policies there may not permit the use of reflexology.

Therapists who are not midwives should also be ultra-cautious in treating women whose labour is beginning to deviate from normal, for example when uterine action is uncoordinated, the fetal head remains high above the pelvic brim or the fetal position is posterior (see Chapter 5). If the uterus becomes hypertonic the non-midwife therapist should refrain from giving any treatment. Similarly, in the event of delay in either the second or third stages of labour, or if there is bleeding or an atonic uterus immediately post delivery, the therapist should have a discussion with the midwife to determine the exact cause of the delay and should only provide RZT if s/he fully understands the physio-pathological basis of the mother's condition. In the event of any fetal distress, no treatment should be given at all.

Table 2.2 Contraindications and precautions to reflex zone therapy in pregnancy, birth and puerperium

	Absolute contraindications	Precautions
General	Maternal preference	Immediately post-operatively
	Professional doubt	Medication, depends on medical condition
	Deep vein thrombosis	Foot conditions – verrucae, corns, athlete's
	Pulmonary embolism	foot, eczema
	Pyrexia	Phlebitis
	Foot fracture	Carcinoma
	Amputation	Gallstones
	Active arthritis affecting feet	Renal calculi
	Epilepsy	Intra-uterine contraceptive device
	Cardiac conditions	Psychiatric illness
	Systemic infections	Addictions
Pregnancy	IVF – whilst taking ovulatory	Preconception period
	stimulants	Sub-fertility
	IVF – once fertilised blastocyst	First trimester
	re-implanted	History of miscarriage in previous pregnancy
	Threatened miscarriage	Anti-hypertensives
	Cervical suture in situ	Thyroid medication
	Anticoagulants	Diet-controlled diabetes
	Non-steroidal anti-inflammatory	Mild hypertension or pre-eclampsia
	drugs	Grade 1 or 2 placenta praevia in 3rd trimester
	Insulin-dependent diabetes	Iron deficiency anaemia
	mellitus	Excess Braxton Hicks
	Fulminating pre-eclampsia	Preterm membrane rupture
	History of eclampsia	Intrauterine growth retardation
	Active vaginal bleeding	Twins
	Grade 3 or 4 placenta praevia	Grande multiparity (4+)
	Sickle cell anaemia or other	
	haematological disorders	
	Post-operatively	
	Threatened preterm labour	
	Reduced fetal movements	
	Triplets, quadruplets	
	Extreme grande multiparity (7+)	
Labour	Preterm labour	Abnormal uterine action
	Induction techniques before term	Abnormal presentation
	With epidural	High presenting part
		Delay in first, second or third stage
		With other analgesia
Puerperium	Thrombo-embolic disorders	Slow uterine involution or excessive lochia

> **Box 2.3** Stages of reflex zone treatment
>
> - Assessment – comprehensive, relevant history
> - Inspection of the feet to aid in making a decision about treatment requirements
> - Manual palpation of the feet, using the special grip technique and the preferred treatment sequence, combined with appropriate specific techniques to stimulate or sedate relevant reflex zones
> - After care advice and record keeping
> - Evaluation and follow-up

In the immediate postnatal period, general relaxation treatments can be given daily in order to facilitate adaption to parenthood and to establish breast feeding and a return of the mother's body to the non-pregnant state, but caution should be employed in the event of any signs or symptoms of infection or thrombo-embolic conditions. If the midwife believes from clinical signs that the mother has a poorly involuting uterus or excessive lochial discharges, the uterine points on the feet should not be stimulated, to avoid the possibility of torrential haemorrhage from retained products of conception.

REFLEX ZONE THERAPY TREATMENT SEQUENCE

Inspection of the feet

The mother should be informed that the hands-on part of the treatment session commences with a visual examination of the feet. The practitioner should take into account *any* visible irregularities and make a note of them, as they may be significant. It is not *appropriate* to soak the feet in warm water, either to wash them or for relaxation, immediately prior to treatment, as warmth will distort the inspection and palpation elements of the treatment. The two feet should be examined, in a good light, *without touching*, for uniformity. The non-touch procedure is essential to avoid stretching the skin which can interfere with visibility of minor irregularities in the feet.

When examining the feet, it is necessary to observe the variations between the two feet of the individual, as well as relating these to what is known about feet in general; an aspect of RZT which improves with experience. Note the position of the two feet on the couch. The feet may be seen to point at different angles, or the two heels may come to rest with one further down the couch than the other, suggesting that the two sides of the body are out of line, in keeping with the theoretical basis of structural RZT. It is useful also to take into account any apparent differences between the left and right sides of the body, which may be implied by aspects other than on the feet. For example, note how evenly the woman's top rests on her shoulders; irregularities may be observed if one side of the blouse reveals more of one shoulder than the other, or if a necklace appears to be resting unevenly on the clavicle bones. A belt may sit on the hips at a tilted angle (although this may, of course, be a conscious fashion statement), or the two pockets on a pair of jeans may be seen to be at different levels. These variations may reflect a "lop-sided" pelvis, perhaps due to previous trauma, disease or genetic influences, but which may also indirectly affect internal organs as a result of the strain and tension placed on one side of the body. Similarly, impressions on the feet made by shoes may be seen and should not be dismissed purely as indentations from tight shoes. Where a pressure area is more pronounced on one foot than the other, this again may relate to an imbalance between the two sides of the body.

Much has been made of "reading" the feet, although there is no research to support a somewhat esoteric interpretation of personality traits. An unproven example is that the right foot is said to represent the past life and masculine traits, while the left represents the present life and feminine traits. However, without doubt, experiential observations do intimate a close correlation with certain claims made by non-academic experts. For example, tension and rigidity in the feet is thought to correspond to a generalised tension throughout the body and/or mind. A long big (first) toe, the reflex zone for the head and neck, usually indicates a long neck, whereas people with a short neck often have short, stumpy first toes. A high foot arch, the reflex zone for the spine, may indicate a noticeable sacral curve in the lower back. Cyclical puffiness on the dorsum, just below the toes, in the area corresponding to the reflex zone for the breast, can be seen when a woman is pre-menstrual and suffering swollen, tender breasts. Notice whether the feet curve inwards (said to represent an introspective personality), point outwards (an outgoing personality) or stand upright (an organised, rigid personality), which may give an indication of tension, relaxation or anxiety (a "holding back" from the therapist). Note the shape of the feet and each toe, and their relative relationship to one another. For example, where the fifth (little) toe, and sometimes the fourth also, bend under the edge of the foot, this may suggest shoulder or clavicle misalignment, as the bony edge of the foot is the reflex zone for the shoulder. Webbing between the toes, the zone for the lymphatics to the head and neck, could be a sign of congestion in this area, leading to the possibility of idiopathic recurrent headaches. (See Stormer 2007 for more on this aspect of reflexology.)

The feet should be examined for any fluctuations in colour. Whilst large areas of pigmentation change will be easily seen, the trained eye may notice more precise and localised changes, with a variety of hues, ranging from pink to red, white, yellow, orange, brown, black, grey, blue and even areas with "green" tinges. These may or may not be significant, but some common colour irregularities occur with specific conditions. Examples include: a deepening orange hue on the inner heel as pregnancy progresses, in the zone related to the uterus and a darkening grey–brown colour beneath the lower half of the inner ankle bone, which corresponds to the zone for the symphysis pubis, when pubic discomfort is present or symphysis pubis diastasis is developing in late pregnancy. Linear flecks or areas of apparent pressure on the feet may relate to the site of scars, either from trauma or from surgery. For example, a low suprapubic incision for minor gynaecological surgery such as a laparotomy may leave a thin line visible on the dorsal surface of one or both feet, approximately at the point where a sandal strap would rest. This is the reflex zone area for the base of the abdominal musculature, merging into the reflex zone for the fallopian tube and pelvic lymphatics.

Similarly, the location of any small areas of infection, verrucae, corns, warts, eczema or dermatitis, should be noted. These usually correspond to the reflex zone representing the causative areas of the body relative to the presenting condition or they may indicate past medical conditions, or occasionally presage developing conditions. The temperature of the feet should also be noted both at the beginning and at various stages during and after the treatment; there is commonly a noticeable difference between the first and second foot being treated.

Obvious irregularities such as foot and ankle oedema will be seen immediately, but it is also important to recognise any variations in the skin, perhaps in the form of pitting, dips, crevasses, bulges or bulbous areas. Additionally, the elasticity of the skin should be observed, another indication of the overall health of the feet and of the body. Their significance will be dependent on the exact location on the feet and the reflex zone to which this area relates. Note if the skin is firm or flaccid, dry and flaky, well nourished and smooth, or even sweaty and moist. Towards term pregnant women frequently have extremely dry skin around the bases of the heels, a fact which may simply be due to their altered centre of gravity as abdominal size increases. However, this area is also the reflex zone for the pelvic organs, which are obviously working hard at this time and it is interesting to postulate as to whether this has a reflexology-associated significance. Other patches of dry or flaking skin may be even more significant depending on where they are situated. Marquardt (2000:191) comments on the appearance of fine beads of moisture which appear on the feet of pregnant women who are anxious or stressed, usually found on the inner sides of the two heels, the areas for the reflex zones to the uterus.

It is essential not to omit the visual inspection, especially at the first appointment, as this can contribute greatly to the overall assessment prior to a specific treatment. Whilst inspection alone does not provide an adequate means of diagnosis, it is a valuable adjunct to the booking and pre-treatment history aspects of the assessment. It is interesting that the feet sometimes reveal conditions which the mother may not have admitted to or may have forgotten when the booking history is being taken by the midwife. For example, the teeth zones on the sides of the toes are often tender during pregnancy but, rather than necessarily indicating the need for dental fillings it may relate to sore and bleeding gums which are common antenatally.

Box 2.4 Observation of the feet prior to the manual component of reflex zone therapy treatment

- Position and angle of each foot; differences between feet
- Situation of the two feet on the couch
- Relationship of each toe to the others
- Colour variations, patches, flecks and spots of colour
- Textural variations – dips, swellings, etc.
- Irregularities and infections
- Skin conditions

Manual palpation of the feet

Reflexology – and in particular RZT – is *not* simply a foot massage, although it may incorporate aspects of massage for the relaxation part of the treatment. Most treatments will commence with some stroking, manipulation of the bony areas of the feet, holding, stretching and other techniques which contribute to a sense of relaxation in the woman; some of these may be repeated towards the end of treatment, together with other movements which bring the session to a conclusion (see Suggested treatment sequence, Appendix 1). It is also acceptable to incorporate some of the effleurage and petrissage movements of massage, either during or at the end of the treatment to reinforce the relaxation effect.

The practitioner's thumbs and fingers then undertake a thorough exploration of the woman's feet, working over the entire surface of both feet and covering all reflex zones. This may be followed, if appropriate, by treatment of specific points which have been identified during this exploratory stage. A particular grip is used, in which the tip of the working digit travels over the surface of the feet with a movement which can be likened to a "caterpillar crawling". Initially, practitioners use their dominant thumb to perfect this technique, whilst the other fingers support the foot. Once proficient, this technique can then be extended to the opposite thumb and the fingers of both hands. The bent thumb is positioned on the foot so that the tip presses inwards slightly, then straightens and slides, without losing contact, in a minimal movement to the next millimetre of the surface of the foot. This rhythmic *"indent – straighten – slide"* movement forms the basis of the initial exploration of the feet.

The exploring thumb or finger tip must become sensitive to nuances in the feet that may indicate the need for specific sedation or stimulation of relevant reflex zones. The practitioner may feel variations which alert her to underlying conditions, which may or may not have been mentioned by the mother. These may feel like grains of sand, sugar or rice beneath the skin in particular areas of the feet, or occasionally a sensation of minute air bubbles under the skin surface. This is a phenomenon that is relatively easily felt on the plantar surface of the feet, at the base of the little (5th) toes in the areas corresponding to the scapulae, because many people have slightly stiff shoulders as a result of their normal day-to-day activities. It was previously believed in generic reflexology that this graininess related to the accumulation of lactic acid crystals, although this theory has now been rejected; however this and other irregularities felt in the feet by the practitioner are thought to represent a build-up of toxins. Sometimes a hard "knot" of tissue is felt, not dissimilar to the "knots" of muscular tension felt by therapists performing full body massage. On other occasions the therapist may feel that the tissues are oedematous, or rigid and resistant to pressure. Sometimes the practitioner will experience a feeling of minute pulsation beneath the examining finger or thumb, which may appear to "buzz" or feel similar to a small electric shock. It is thought that this is a transfer of energy between the therapist and the client, but may also alert a sensitive and intuitive practitioner to areas of the body which may have altered homeostasis.

Specific therapeutic techniques

Once the initial visual and manual assessment has been completed other techniques may be used to treat the presenting condition or any others which have been revealed during the first part of the session. RZT does not take a formulaic approach to treating medical conditions but individualises treatment according to these revelations. However, it is essential to have an underpinning knowledge and understanding of the physiology and potential pathology which may be relevant, in order to determine the most appropriate and safest techniques.

In RZT there are several actions which may be taken as a result of the visual and manual assessments: sedation, stimulation or no action. For generic reflexologists this is sometimes a difficult concept to grasp as they are taught that all treatment, even that for general relaxation, "stimulates" the system and restores or maintains homeostasis. This is probably a matter of semantics, the word "stimulating" actually meaning "facilitating" or "rebalancing". However, the clinical nature of RZT requires the practitioner to identify when specific treatment is required and to act accordingly. It is *not* appropriate to perform the same treatment on each person and it is important to rationalise, in the context of the individual's physiopathology, exactly how to facilitate that return to homeostatic balance. Furthermore, the inclination of generic reflexologists to "massage" any point on the feet in which the client feels discomfort or which the practitioner believes is disordered, is to be discouraged. Inappropriate massage can over-stimulate a reflex point, theoretically exposing the client to the risk of "overdose" and potentially making them ill.

The practitioner must develop an appreciation of the depth of pressure that can be applied to the feet and be able to interpret their implications. The tone of the tissue on the surfaces of the feet alter with thumb or finger pressure, normal tissue returning to its original position by bouncing back immediately the thumb is removed. Women with varying degrees of developing or actual pathology will exhibit a range of tissue reactions which differ from this norm, including "grittiness" beneath the surface of the skin, rigidity, inelasticity, fluidity and deep indentation. All of these may cause discomfort or pain for the woman.

Sedation is performed to suppress an acute symptom, such as pain, usually in response to the client's reporting of sharp tenderness at a precise location on the foot. Long-standing problems usually present with a bruised sensation in the relevant reflex zone, although this can be quite intense and may initially be the sharp or burning sensation which then changes to a deeper but more bearable and sometimes more diversified pain. It will depend on the nature of the tenderness and the possible cause of the problem as to whether sedation is applied precisely over the point or in a more diversified manner. For example, headache in the temples can be eased by applying sedating techniques precisely over the reflex points for the temples, whereas a more generalised headache may better be treated by using a calming pressure over the entire surface of the big toes, to allow for more widespread sedation. Sedation may be required for up to 2 minutes at a time or may need to be performed in stages, according to the mother's tolerance. Normally the practitioner can ask the mother for feedback whilst the technique is performed. The mother may report that the nature of the tenderness changes, indicating the need to release the pressure and repeat the sedation. Often the second phase of sedation will feel more tender to the mother than the first, but as the procedure is repeated several times (usually about five), the tenderness should become less until it no longer is felt in the foot. However, it should not be assumed that maternal reports of acute tenderness always imply the need for sedation of the point; the practitioner must consider the possible cause of this tenderness before attempting any specific treatment. For example, a urinary tract infection may, in reflexology terms, present with acute tenderness felt by the mother in the foot zones for the renal tract. However, whilst sedation may suppress the localised pain, it will do nothing to kill the pathogens and it may, if undertaken without due understanding, exacerbate and spread the infection.

Stimulation would be appropriate for a reflexology point which required a boost to the physiology. Examples would be stimulation to the arches of the feet, the reflex zones for the intestines, to treat constipation, or to increase oxytocin release to aid contractions by stimulating the pituitary zones on the plantar surfaces of the big (1st) toes (*not* the uterine zone). Generalised stimulation is a brisk continuation of the "caterpillar walking" movement, whilst specific stimulation involves applying pressure intermittently to a precise reflex point. Initially the mother may feel no tenderness at the point of stimulation but some discomfort may develop as the procedure continues; it is not the intention to cause the mother excessive pain but, as with sedating techniques, to work only to the level of the mother's tolerance. Importantly, tenderness at specific points on the feet does not always automatically require stimulation – and it is vital that generic reflexologists do not merely start to *massage* or rub the relevant reflex point as this in itself constitutes a form of stimulation which could theoretically exacerbate the client's symptoms.

It can be seen that these two techniques are at opposite ends of the spectrum of therapeutic action and thus need to be used only when appropriate. Determining the correct technique is reliant on a thorough understanding of physiology. By inference, using the wrong technique could exacerbate a symptom or condition, for example stimulating the zone for the head could worsen a headache, whilst sedating the zone for the intestine – or, indeed, stimulating it in the wrong direction – could, theoretically, lead to further constipation, possibly in extreme cases, if one takes it to its logical conclusion, even to impaction of the bowel.

Occasionally it is necessary to note a disordered foot zone, as identified by visual examination or as felt by either the mother or the practitioner, but to take *no specific action*. An example of vital importance in maternity RZT is the pituitary zone. During the antenatal period pituitary hormones are fundamental to the continuance of the pregnancy; therefore, the pituitary reflex zone will be tender throughout. It is not appropriate to stimulate these points as this could potentially trigger contractions, leading either to miscarriage in early pregnancy or to preterm labour in the third trimester. It is also incorrect to sedate these points as this could suppress the release of pituitary hormones, similarly leading to fetal loss. Thus, when treating pregnant women and working over the first toe with the generalised "caterpillar crawling" movement, the examining finger should neither pause nor press strongly on the pituitary zone, the thumb or finger should simply pass across it and on to the next area of the toe. The area should not be totally avoided as this could cause the mother to feel that the treatment was incomplete; gentle stroking and light massage movements can be used as required.

In structural RZT an additional technique is frequently employed – *manipulation*. Although some manipulative techniques are used in both generic reflexology and in RZT, structural RZT relies more heavily on working the zones for the musculoskeletal system, as the therapy is based on the principles of osteopathy (see Chapter 1). In dynamic manipulation the practitioner uses his/her hands to exert a firm yet gentle movement to relevant passive zones of the feet with the intention of mobilising, adjusting and applying traction to influence the bones, ligaments, joints and related nerves of the body. Put simply, structural RZT can be likened to osteopathy, but applied via the reflex zones of the feet. To generic practitioners, basic RZT can sometimes appear to be more forceful than the style to which they are accustomed; structural RZT may appear even more so, especially since it frequently elicits "cracking" noises and sensations from the feet. However, unlike Rwo Shur reflexology, a Taiwanese form used extensively in Asia, in which pressure to specific reflex points is applied exceptionally firmly, structural RZT does not rely on this somewhat indiscriminate pressure. Instead, it focuses on precise manipulative movements based on an understanding of the implications of musculoskeletal misalignment on the individual's overall condition and underpinned by sound theoretical knowledge of the aetiology and differential diagnosis of particular symptoms or conditions.

Table 2.3 Therapeutic techniques in structural reflex zone therapy

Technique	Method	Aim	Features	Cautions
Generalised foot massage	Effleurage (stroking) of feet, with or without oils or creams (no oils if prior to reflex zone therapy [RZT] techniques)	Relaxation, warming of feet, nurturing, starts communication between client and therapist	Should be pleasurable, not painful or ticklish	Firm pressure avoids tickling sensations Normal precautions to massage apply
Holding	Gentle firm pressure on diverse area of foot, e.g. around heel, across all five toes	Nurturing and calming, allows pause in treatment sequence especially if feet are tender	Warm, comforting and pleasurable	Do not prolong hold if precise reflex point
"Sweeping"	Firm bimanual dragging of thumbs across specific area, e.g. diaphragm, around hip zone, along reflex zone for Eustachian tube	Calming, pain relieving, restores homeostasis, aids drainage of fluid	Less tender to touch if zone disordered, can be very calming	Ensure movement is performed in correct direction
Draining	Sweeping movement with forefinger and thumb	Thought to "drain" or encourage improved flow of lymphatics, aids circulation	May cause a "pinching" sensation; repeat 2–3 times to reduce tenderness (normal)	Do not overwork the area – can cause nausea and other strong reactions especially in pregnancy

Continued

Table 2.3	Therapeutic techniques in structural reflex zone therapy—Cont'd			
Technique	Method	Aim	Features	Cautions
"Caterpillar crawling"	Continuous flowing action of thumb/finger over entire surface of foot; two or three fingers can be used together if appropriate	Facilitates exploration of foot for areas requiring further treatment; can be relaxing in itself	Firm but not painful unless passing over an affected zone	Therapist must become alert to *every* nuance in the feet which may indicate other treatment needed
Sedation	Sustained pressure applied to specific point; wait until pain in the point subsides then repeat 4–5 times Sometimes used as a "first aid" technique	Slows specific physiological activity and suppresses symptoms	Tenderness at reflex point gradually subsides – second application may be more tender (normal)	Work only to the level of the client's tolerance
Stimulation	Intermittent pulsation with the thumb or finger for 20–30 presses, 0.5 seconds apart	Accelerates physiological activity – encourages more efficient physical processes	Client may report sharp tenderness at reflex point – may become increasingly tender	Work only to the level of client's tolerance
Manipulation (structural RZT)	Firm working of bony parts of feet	Aids realignment of musculoskeletal system	May be painful; "cracks" and "popping" sensations felt or heard	Be aware of rapid strong reactions Do not force bony resistance
No action	No sedation or stimulation applied to the relevant point	Avoids sedation or stimulation of particular reflex points	Do not omit this area of the foot completely – pass hands across reflex point gently	If in doubt about any other technique – do nothing

Aftercare advice, record keeping and evaluation

As with any other healthcare intervention it is important to provide adequate advice and information to ensure the effectiveness of the treatment and to alert the mother to any side effects which may occur. This can be given both verbally and in writing if necessary. The mother's records should be completed either as a separate set of notes or within the normal handheld maternity notes (see Professional Issues).

The mother should be advised to drink plenty of water for the 24 hours following treatment to flush her system through, as it is believed that reflexology, in common with many other complementary therapies, facilitates the release of toxins which need to be eliminated from the body. She should also be advised to avoid stimulants, such as caffeine in the form of coffee, tea and cola drinks; alcohol; excessive exercise and heavy housework or occupational exertion. Ideally, the mother should be encouraged to relax as much as her personal circumstances permit; she may find that she is surprisingly tired to the point of exhaustion on the day of treatment, especially after the first, and should, if at all possible, go to bed fairly early. She should be warned to be aware of any reactions to the treatment and to report any which worry her unduly (see below).

At the subsequent appointment the practitioner should enquire about the mother's condition following the first treatment, recording any reactions, side effects, concerns, improvements or deteriorations in her general wellbeing. This will enable the therapist to make any necessary adaptations to the treatment and form the basis for ongoing care.

REACTIONS TO TREATMENT

Reactions to RZT during and after treatment are a common and normal phenomenon and are an indication that the body is attempting to harness its own self-healing capacity, ridding itself of toxins and facilitating a return to homeostasis. They should, therefore, not be viewed as "adverse" reactions or side effects, but rather as an indication that the mother's body is responding to the treatment. However, reactions in pregnant women can sometimes be very profound with a rapid onset. The practitioner should observe the mother's reactions carefully (another justification for treating her sitting upright) and may need to pause or cease treatment if her reactions are too marked. In order to give informed consent to treatment she should be advised prior to commencing that these reactions may occur, sometimes during the actual session, or afterwards, both in the short term and the longer term. She should also be encouraged to report *any* apparent reactions, side effects or adverse symptoms which occur between treatments.

As the practitioner works over the surfaces of the feet during a treatment session the mother may report feeling various sensations in response. These include tenderness, usually either a sharp, almost burning sensation or a deep bruised feeling. It is vital to encourage her to report these as the treatment session proceeds, as they may have a bearing on the subsequent specific techniques employed (see above). It is this aspect of RZT which requires the two-way interaction between therapist and client and means that, at this stage, she is not merely a passive recipient. The tender area of the foot may not always appear to be the same as that which relates to the history, but may enable the therapist to differentiate between *symptomatic* and *causative* zones of the feet. For example, the mother may complain of backache in the sacrum yet RZT palpation suggests that the cause of the backache is more thoracic than sacral. It is *not* appropriate for the novice to attempt to "massage" any of these areas until more definitive assessment has been undertaken to facilitate an understanding of the precise nature of the problem, which may then indicate whether stimulation or sedation of the reflex zone, or another technique, is necessary.

Physiological reactions may develop in response to the physical effects of the treatment; for example localised and systemic changes in body temperature, including feeling hot, becoming clammy and perspiring, or, conversely, feeling cold and starting to shiver or shake. This may be accompanied by changes in skin colour, such as redness or pallor of the face or feet. These reactions are thought to occur as a result of stimulating the reflex zones for the systemic nervous system, leading to tachycardia, pupil dilatation, respiratory alterations, perspiration, dry mouth and localised erythema or pallor from increased spleen activity.

Pregnant women also frequently experience emotional effects during and after treatment and may burst into tears or start giggling uncontrollably. This type of reaction is often preceded by changes in facial expression, such as grimacing or smiling, or by gestures, including clenching of the fists, tweaking of the clothing or waving of the hands. Often the latter is in response to the discomfort which can be felt during certain aspects of the treatment, as when the practitioner focuses on a relevant reflex zone that elicits tenderness or pain in the feet. Sometimes the mother will report more significant reactions including nausea (although vomiting is rare), a desire to urinate or palpitations. In addition, stimulation of specific reflex points on the feet can trigger feelings of dizziness and light-headedness. This is particularly pertinent to pressure applied to the relaxation point (formerly named the "solar plexus" reflex point, see Chapter 3) and practitioners should always work on this point very lightly when treating pregnant women.

Depending on the response and the severity of sensations, it may be appropriate to stop the treatment, even if only temporarily, and to use gentle sedating and calming techniques, such as simple stroking and holding of the feet. If the practitioner considers that continuation of the treatment may be possible it is important to retain contact with the feet so that some degree of continuity can be maintained. Again, depending on the precise reactions, the mother may require a cold or warm drink, tissues, blanket, vomit bowl or a visit to the bathroom. All responses to treatment should be recorded and the practitioner should analyse their techniques to determine if any particular aspect of the session contributed to an exacerbation of the reactions. If possible, the mother should be given the opportunity to rest before leaving the treatment area – either in the same room, another room or in the waiting area.

Other reactions may occur within the first 24 hours following treatment or occasionally later; although they are most often after the first treatment, they may re-emerge or change in response to a course of treatments.Normally the reactions subside after 24 to 48 hours. The majority of women report a sense of overall relaxation and a good night's sleep on the day of the treatment, although some experience vivid dreams (more than the normal memories of dreaming which are common in pregnancy), sometimes to the extent of fearsome nightmares. Whilst initially the mother may feel exhausted or lethargic immediately after treatment, this is usually followed by an increase in energy, enabling them to cope with their symptoms better. It is, however, important to advise the mother of the possibility of this reaction, and to warn her not to use it as a misguided opportunity to "catch up" on all the things she has postponed whilst feeling unwell or in pain, as this will only serve to exacerbate or complicate her presenting symptoms or cause a relapse.

Minor reactions include skin changes such as redness, temporary eczema or eruptions, such as spots, as well as increased perspiration which may be malodorous. Many women report increased micturition which is often slightly malodorous and with sediment, so the practitioner should be aware of that which is a normal response to RZT and that which may indicate a urinary tract infection. Changes in the frequency of defaecation and the amount and consistency of stools, sometimes with added mucus, may also occur, and the mother may report increased flatulence. Similarly, increased mucus production in the nasal passages is common, leading to nasal dripping, sinus congestion or catarrh. Headaches, backache or other aches and pains may arise, reflecting either old injuries or the secondary sites of metabolic waste which has not been excreted via the normal channels. A heavier-than-normal vaginal discharge may also develop, but the practitioner should ensure that this is not indicative of a gestational vaginal infection. In non-pregnant clients the next menstrual period may occur prematurely, may be heavier than normal and be of a different consistency and colour. Some women experience increased lacrimation, discharge from the ears or mouth ulcers. Scars from old wounds may become irritable and itch more than normal.

Most commonly women seeking treatment for specific pregnancy conditions report a slight worsening of their symptoms for 24 to 48 hours. This is a "healing crisis" which is a normal feature of many complementary therapies including RZT, homeopathy and osteopathy. It is usually a prelude to improvement in the client's general condition (rather than a side effect of the treatment), brought about by the body attempting to expel toxic factors which have caused or contributed to the condition for which treatment was requested, and to trigger the healing process. Advice should be given about how to deal with this, either through rest and recuperation, relevant dietary or exercise strategies or, occasionally, a temporary use of pharmacological analgesics, although this should be avoided where possible to prevent further toxicity due to drug metabolism in the liver. Furthermore, some women report the recurrence of symptoms related to old injuries or medical conditions, for example discomfort in a part of the body where there have been previous fractures. This is temporary and normal, being an holistic reaction of the body to RZT, as opposed to merely a reductionist reaction in that part of the body currently affected. The mother should be reassured that these reactions are normal. Future treatment options will depend on the intensity of the healing crisis, indicating whether the treatment should be continued, adapted or stopped.

Adaptations may be required during the next treatment session if the post-treatment reactions are severe; the most likely being to shorten the duration of the session or to lighten the depth of manual pressure on the feet. Pregnant women may not be able to endure a traditional full-length treatment (approximately an hour) and it is wise to keep standard antenatal RZT sessions to a maximum of 35 minutes' duration. If a course of treatment is in progress it may be useful to decrease the frequency of sessions. In any case RZT should not be performed on expectant mothers more than once in every 3–5 days; treatment intended solely for relaxation purposes should not be undertaken more than once a week. If the time between treatments is short, the mother's body does not have time to react to the previous session, nor to recover from any responses which cause her discomfort. It is very easy to "overdose" any client and particularly those who are pregnant.

Table 2.4 Reactions to treatment	
Reactions during treatment	Reactions after treatment
Tenderness in feet – sharp, burning	Relaxation/energised
Tenderness in feet – dull, bruise-like	Tiredness/sleep well
Pain in relevant/distal area of body	Disturbed sleep/vivid dreams
Facial expressions, gestures	Skin changes/eruptions
Temperature changes – hot, clammy, perspiring	Increased diuresis, malodorous urine
Temperature changes – cold, shivering	Increased defaecation, malodorous stools
Muscle contractions, shaking	Increased sweating, lacrimation, nasal
Colour changes – feet or body	discharge, vaginal discharge
Nausea, vomiting	Mood changes
Desire to pass urine	Exacerbation of presenting symptoms
Palpitations, dizziness	Re-emergence of old symptoms
Emotional outbursts – crying, laughing	No apparent reaction

Very occasionally women have no reaction to RZT at all, especially after the first treatment session. This is usually when the mother's condition is particularly severe, particularly in cases of musculoskeletal problems such as symphysis pubis discomfort or sciatica, and she may require several treatments to obtain any relief. However, a record should be made of the fact that no reaction has yet occurred and the practitioner should expect the mother to have a healing crisis response following another one or two treatments.

3

Reflex zones used in structural reflex zone therapy for maternity care

Before considering specific reflex zone treatment of pregnant, labouring and newly delivered mothers it is necessary to become familiar with the precise reflex zones of the feet and the various types of treatment for safe practice. Whilst this chapter is aimed primarily at midwives with little previous knowledge of RZT, it will also serve as a reminder to therapists who practise generic reflexology and may challenge some of their previously held views about the therapy, particularly in relation to treating pregnant clients.

There are many different charts or maps used in the various styles of reflexology, and there remains considerable disagreement amongst reflexology authorities regarding the precise location of several reflex points, notably the "solar plexus", pituitary gland, liver, knees, rectum and anus. Unfortunately, these inconsistencies, although potentially encouraging academic debate, do little to improve the credibility of reflexology amongst sceptical medical colleagues and while they persist it is unlikely that reflexology will achieve full recognition from the conventional healthcare establishment. However, increasing popularity and use of the therapy provides considerable amounts of experiential evidence, initiating debate which may contribute to further development of the therapy. Until more is understood regarding the mechanism of action and the physiological underpinning of reflexology, theory and practice will continue to vary between one school of thought and another and will need to be based on "best practice" by experienced and knowledgeable practitioners, and on treatments which are both safe and effective.

It is this notion of "best practice" that may influence future thinking, initiate debate and lead to consolidation of theoretical principles. In the same way as the anatomy of the breast has recently been found to vary from our original traditional thinking (Medela 2006), so too will zones and reflex points on the feet, especially as it becomes an increasingly clinical modality rather than merely a form of relaxation therapy. The profession of generic reflexology, in common with other complementary therapies, is evolving into a range of specialist clinical areas, in which therapists develop enhanced awareness and advanced practice pertinent to varying clinical fields, for example palliative care or learning disability care. Maternity care is also a clinical specialty in its own right. Although there is now a requirement under the reflexology core curriculum that all training programmes include reproductive health at the pre-qualifying level, it is vital that therapists acknowledge the specific needs of expectant mothers and the *risks* of performing reflexology without adequate understanding on this client group.

This chapter covers the reflex points of direct relevance when treating pregnant and childbearing women. An approach is used in this chapter which introduces first those reflex zones most relevant to maternity care, and builds up to a complete picture appropriate for treating pregnant women. There are some points which have not been discussed in depth, as these do not normally have any direct bearing on maternity RZT, although they will, of course, be treated during a general relaxation session encompassing the "caterpillar crawling" movement over the entire surfaces of both feet.

The differences in the locations of reflex zones detailed in this book may be due to the variations between generic reflexology and RZT. Occasionally, readers will observe differences of opinion between this book and other RZT authorities, but zone location here is based on the results of over 20 years' experience and the treatment of well over 5000 pregnant and childbearing women undertaken by this author. It is felt that, where variations exist, the zones used here may, in fact, be *indirect* zones for an organ or body part, rather than a direct zone, but are those which, in practice, appear to achieve the best results and will, therefore, be referred to as *working zones*. Readers may also wish to refer to one of the principal textbooks on RZT to complete their knowledge of all the body zones and points (for example, Lett 2000, Marquardt 2000), whilst bearing in mind the variations between authorities.

RELAXATION POINTS

The diaphragm

It is useful first to locate the reflex zone for the diaphragm for relaxation purposes, and as an aid to the accurate location of other zones, since this is one of the dividing lines between the transverse zone for the thorax and that for the abdomen. It is found on the plantar surface of the foot and, like its anatomical counterpart, is a thin line between the zones for the lungs and the abdominal cavity. If we consider that on the sole or plantar surface the ball of the foot represents the zone for the lungs and the arch of the foot is the zone for the intestines, the diaphragm naturally falls between the two. The point at which the ball and the arch of the foot are differentiated by a colour and textural change represents the diaphragm zone (see Figs 3.1, 3.5).

A deep sense of relaxation can be achieved by "diaphragm sweeping", in which the practitioner places his/her two thumb pads on the relaxation point

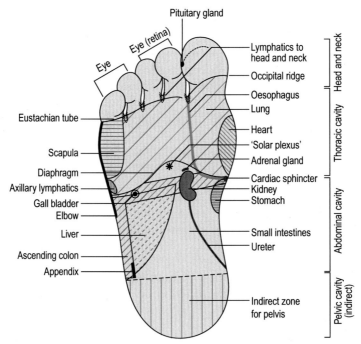

Fig. 3.1 Reflex zones on the sole (right)

("solar plexus") zone immediately under the diaphragm line, then firmly and slowly sweeps outwards with both thumbs simultaneously to the distal edges of the feet. This can be repeated twice more, then on the other foot, and is a particularly good technique for current stress, whereas the "solar plexus" point is effective in relieving the immediate physiological effects of longer-term stress and the adrenal gland zones are used only for acute stress and panic (see below).

The relaxation point ("solar plexus")

The primary relaxation point (formerly called the "solar plexus") is an example of a point which is not logically sited, even in traditional reflexology charts. The "solar plexus" refers to the sympathetic nerves and ganglia in the peritoneal cavity, with branches which supply nerves to the abdominal viscera. This corresponds to the central area just below the xiphisternum and diaphragm, where one may experience a sensation of "butterflies" when nervous. In conventional medical terminology, it is now more commonly known as the *coeliac* plexus, the largest autonomic nerve centre in the body, located in the abdomen behind the stomach and in front of the aorta. Neural branches assist in controlling a variety of vital body functions including adrenal secretion and intestinal contraction.

It has already been stated that the two feet represent a "map" of the whole body, with the left foot relating to the left side of the body and the right foot to the right side. The dorsum of the foot represents the front of the body, the plantar surfaces correspond to the internal organs and the midline of the body is represented by the inner aspects of the feet. Logic demands that, since the two feet placed together represent the two halves of the body, the "solar plexus" point should be situated in the medial section of each foot, i.e. in zone 1. However, tradition has placed this reflex point in the central area of *each* plantar surface of the feet, i.e. in zone 3. The majority of reflexology texts continue to site the so-called "solar plexus" point in zone 3 of each foot (and some consumer websites were found on the internet which located it, inaccurately, in zone 2). On balance, however, it is probably more accurate to refer to this as the "relaxation point", which coincidentally corresponds to the acupuncture point Kidney 1, the first point on the Kidney meridian, also used for relaxation. One early text (Lambert 1988:42) positioned the solar plexus in zone 1 and Marquardt (2000:73) has changed her location to zone 1, having previously placed it in zone 3 (1983:52); although Lett (2000:168,169) has not made this adjustment.

Locating the "relaxation point" requires the plantar surface of the foot to be easily visible with the big toe placed perpendicularly – pointing directly up – towards the ceiling. Drawing an imaginary line down from the tip of the third toe, move down the ball of the foot, until reaching the zone for the diaphragm (see above). Immediately below the diaphragm line is the relaxation point (see Figs 3.1, 3.5). Care should be taken to ensure that the practitioner's finger or thumb is precisely on the reflex point and not overlapping onto the area above the diaphragm line. On the hands, the reflex zone for the relaxation point is in the centre of the palm, in zone 3, at the deepest point when the hand is held as if trying to retain a few drops of water. This can be a useful point in circumstances where the mother's feet are less accessible, for example when the mother is having blood taken in the antenatal clinic.

In pregnant and labouring women it is comparatively easy to over-stimulate the relaxation point, particularly on the feet. They may experience rapid and profound reactions, feeling dizzy, hot or cold, shaky and nauseous. Many reflexology schools teach students to press firmly with a sustained or intermittent pressure on this point in order to achieve a sense of deep relaxation in the client. However, in pregnant mothers, pressure should be applied *extremely lightly* (no more than a touch, with no visible indentation from pressure) and the woman should be observed for adverse reactions (as opposed to normal responses, see Chapter 2) – a justification for treating her sitting upright. This gentle touch should be sustained for no longer than 10 seconds in the first instance until the therapist has observed the mother's response. Stronger reactions are more likely to occur as pregnancy progresses and in labour, as well as in those with obstetric or related medical complications; therefore, this cautious approach is required with each treatment.

Other zones which can be used for relaxation and for specific stress and panic include the lungs and adrenal glands: these are discussed in the relevant sections below.

PITUITARY GLAND

It is absolutely imperative that midwives and reflexologists intending to treat pregnant and childbearing women are able to locate the *most appropriate* point corresponding to the pituitary gland, in order to work safely and to achieve the most effective results from the treatment. The pituitary zone is almost more important to maternity RZT than the zone for the uterus, since it is the "power house" for many aspects of reproductive physiology. The pituitary is, however, perhaps the most difficult point to locate, not least because there are disagreements between authorities, but also because it is such a precise point which is not always easy to see or to feel on the toes. Furthermore, the location differs in every single woman and often between the two feet of the same person.

In the gross anatomy of the human body, the pituitary gland is situated centrally in the middle cranial fossa of the brain, approximately level with the top of the eyes, with the hypothalamus immediately superior to it. Thus, it logically infers that the pituitary gland and hypothalamus reflex points should be found in zone *one* on the medial plantar surface of the big (first) toes. The time may now be right, perhaps, to consider teaching a change of location of the pituitary gland zone from its traditional position, in the same way as the location of the coeliac ("solar") plexus has been altered in recent years. However, it is of interest that, although both Marquardt (2000:39) and Lett (2000) have changed the coeliac plexus location to zone 1, they have retained the position of the pituitary gland zone in the centre of the plantar surface of the large (first) toe. This is usually said to be at the most prominent point of the plantar surface and appears to be the location quoted in the majority of standard reflexology texts. Some authorities in generic reflexology, including Crane (1997) and Dougans (2006), refer to the location as being at the centre of the whorls of the big toes, although Dougans (2006:189) acknowledges that the reflex point is often "off-centre". Interestingly, Enzer is one of very few authors to locate the pituitary in zone 1, and attributes the traditional pituitary location to being the hypothalamus; yet this also defies logic (Enzer 2000:2–22).

On the other hand, this author has found, through many years' experience of using RZT on pregnant women that the zone *most appropriate* to achieving pituitary-related effects appears to be placed *distally* to the midline on the plantar surface of the big toes. Lett (2000:143) and Marquardt (2000:38) both identify this as the temporal lobe of the brain, which is logical, despite a continued illogical positioning of the pituitary gland zone. An Internet search revealed only one style of reflexology, Japanese Ashitsubo, incorporating acupressure points, which sometimes sited the pituitary reflex zone nearer to the distal edge of the plantar surface, whilst the area traditionally identified as the pituitary zone is taken as the point for the cerebrum. However, there was no consistency between the web entries and this would seem to be an unreliable ally for relocating the pituitary zone to the distal surface.

No logical reasoning, in gross anatomical terms, can be given by this author for identifying the pituitary gland reflex zone as being on the distal edge of the big toes. However, anecdotal experience and clinical research undertaken in RZT have shown that this point achieves optimum clinical results in terms of relevant obstetric effects. The point, therefore, probably reflects an indirect or working zone which, for the purposes of maternity RZT, may be safer than attempting to locate the precise *direct* point on the medial aspect of the big toe. It should, however, be noted that the traditional location in the centre of each big toe, is no longer academically appropriate, and further investigation and debate is necessary to determine precisely and universally the location of the pituitary gland points. On the other hand, practitioners who see no justification for changing their practice and who wish to retain the traditional location of the pituitary gland zone should be careful when working over the distal surface of the big toes, since this may cause inadvertent stimulation of the indirect zone.

To locate the pituitary gland reflex zone (the working zone as used in this book) it is vital to visualise the feet in a good light and, initially, for the practitioner to keep his/her hands off the feet completely. It is easiest to define the precise location by drawing an imaginary "y" shape on the plantar surface of the big toe, demarcated by the textural changes which occur. Note first where the big toe rests against the second toe; often the distal surface will be slightly flattened and the skin may be whitish in colour. This forms the upright part of the "y" shape. Next, identify the different skin texture between that part of the big toe which rests on the ground when walking and the tip, which may point slightly upwards in the shoe – this forms one arm of the "y". Then notice the other arm of the "y" where the big toe deviates away from the second toe. The point at which the upright section and the two arms of the "y" meet is the (indirect) location of the pituitary gland reflex zone and provides the most appropriate "working" point. Often a small reddish indentation or a pin-point white dot may be observed, although the presence of this white dot should not be taken automatically as the correct location without further exploration to ascertain the precise point (see Figs 3.1, 3.5).

During RZT that is performed for general relaxation in pregnancy, *no stimulation or sedation* (see Chapter 2) should be applied to the pituitary point – stimulation would increase the output of pituitary hormones, theoretically risking the early onset of uterine contractions, whilst sedation would suppress the essential functioning of the pituitary. On the other hand, the area should not be omitted from a general relaxation treatment but the therapist should merely pass across the point without undertaking any specific action. It is *completely inappropriate* to perform a circular massage of the pituitary reflex zone in pregnancy without justification, as this constitutes a form of stimulation. When it is deemed appropriate to palpate the identified point, use the thumb pad on the opposite hand so that pressure is applied directly to the pituitary point and not diversified over a wider area of skin. If the pressure is applied to the precise location, the woman will feel a slight tenderness, which is sometimes quite sharp, depending on the stage of the menstrual cycle.

REPRODUCTIVE ORGANS

In RZT the reflex zones for the reproductive tract logically reflect the position of these organs within the body, the ovaries being on the distal side of the heels and the uterus being in the midline, divided between the two feet; the fallopian tube joins the ovary zone to the uterus zone. For completeness, the breasts (mammary glands) have also been included here.

Ovaries

To locate the ovary it is useful for the novice to imagine an angle of 90° around the outer aspect of the heel, then to identify the outer ankle bone. Next, imagine a line of 45° dissecting the right angle of the heel, and directed towards the outer ankle bone. The ovary zone is found approximately halfway between the right angle of the heel and the outer ankle bone. In some women this point may be slightly more or slightly less than halfway along this imaginary line; lightly passing a finger across the line will enable the intuitive practitioner to identify the correct point as it may feel like a very small grain of rice and is sometimes visible, especially when active (see Fig. 3.2).

The non-pregnant woman will often feel tenderness, sometimes more in one ovary zone than the other, which experience suggests indicates the active ovary for the current menstrual cycle. As the menstrual cycle progresses from

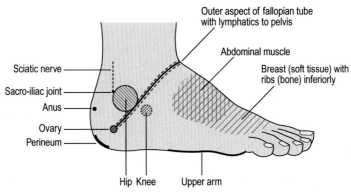

Fig. 3.2   Reflex zones on the lateral (outer) aspect of the foot (right)

menstruation to ovulation the reflex point for the ovary will become more tender, may be more palpable and may be visible as a small red dot on the foot. The point usually remains tender for the duration of the menstrual cycle until menstruation commences. In a woman with polycystic ovary syndrome the practitioner may feel varying degrees of "lumpiness" in one or both ovary zones, which may cause discomfort to the client and which reflect the cystic nature of follicular development within the ovaries. In pregnancy the palpable mass of the ovary zone usually stabilises and equalises on both sides, neither increasing nor decreasing in size.

Uterus

Locating the uterus zone is similar to locating that for the ovary, but is found on the inner aspect of the foot. It can be found approximately one-half to two-thirds of the way towards the ankle bone (it differs on each person) and is usually felt as a dip over the flattened inner edge of the calcaneum, which in some women may be visible. This dip actually represents the fundus and cavity or body of the uterus and in healthy non-pregnant women will normally be the same colour as the surrounding skin of the foot (Fig. 3.3).

During pregnancy the uterus zone changes colour, usually becoming darker, and often taking on an orange hue towards term. As with the pituitary gland zones, the uterus zones should be *neither stimulated nor sedated during pregnancy* unless there is a valid indication to do so. It is interesting also to note here that, in female (non-pregnant) clients who have had a hysterectomy, a larger, more significant dip will be felt, which may feel tender to the woman, usually a deep bruised sensation which may be more intense if the woman continues to experience discomfort from post-surgical adhesions. Irregular "lumpiness" may be felt in this zone in the presence of fibroids; *no* stimulation should be applied if fibroids are suspected, even in non-pregnant clients, as this could cause more severe intermenstrual bleeding and menorrhagia than the woman may already be suffering.

Many reflexologists who treat pregnant women claim that they can determine against which side of the mother's uterus the fetal back is positioned, and this is certainly possible in some women. Unfortunately, reflexologists often misinterpret an appearance of a slightly larger zone on the right foot

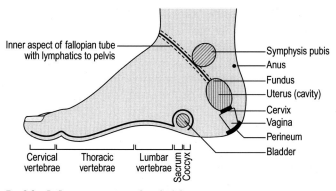

Inner aspect of fallopian tube with lymphatics to pelvis — Symphysis pubis — Anus — Fundus — Uterus (cavity) — Cervix — Vagina — Perineum — Bladder

Cervical vertebrae   Thoracic vertebrae   Lumbar vertebrae   Sacrum   Coccyx

Fig. 3.3   Reflex zones on inner foot (right)

towards term as implying that the fetal back is on the right side, but this actually reflects the right obliquity and rotundity of the uterine anatomy that occurs as pregnancy progresses: towards term, the enlarged uterus is displaced towards the right where there is more space in the abdominal cavity, away from the stomach and slightly rotates to the right on its own axis. On the other hand, an experienced therapist may indeed be able to see or feel a thin firm line on the uterine zone of one foot, which, if the mother is examined abdominally as part of her normal antenatal appointment, may coincide with the midwife's findings regarding the fetal position. It is also possible, occasionally, when gently palpating the uterus zones on the two feet, to feel a small firm round bulge at one end of the zone, which appears to represent the fetal head, and thus one surmises that it could theoretically be possible to determine a cephalic or breech presentation (but *not* to turn the breech to cephalic, see Chapter 5). Very occasionally a minute sliver of red can be seen on one uterine zone, which appears to approximate to the shape of the placenta; accuracy of this finding can be confirmed by referring to the ultrasound scan report for placental location.

The peritoneum, the sheet of tissue which drapes over the pelvic organs and keeps them separate from the abdominal organs, dips down between the bladder and uterus anteriorly (the uterovesical pouch) and between the uterus and rectum posteriorly (the pouch of Douglas). Although it would be difficult to locate the entire reflex zone for the peritoneum, it is useful to be able to locate the zones for these two pouches; tenderness in one or the other, especially post delivery, may indicate the presence of a haematoma or an abscess.

The cervix

The uterine cervix anatomically lies below the cavity of the uterus and forms a canal with an internal and external os (opening). In maternity reflexology, location of the cervix can be useful in certain circumstances during labour, but should only be worked by midwives, or by reflexologists who *fully* understand the relevant physiology and any specific pathology and who can fully justify their decisions either to stimulate or sedate the point (see Chapter 5).

For the purposes of learning to locate the cervix the student therapist should place a finger tip gently on the dip representing the zone for the cavity of the uterus and then slide it down slowly towards the right angle of the heel until a hard ridge is felt. This is a *minute*, almost imperceptible, movement and is only performed as an aid to learning (on non-pregnant models), to enable the student to differentiate between the soft area for the uterine cavity and the hard ridge for the cervix. It can be quite difficult to recognise this ridge but it is important not to keep repeating the downwards movement in an attempt to feel the cervical zone, as this could theoretically trigger problems such as placental separation. If the student is practising on non-pregnant women (which is advisable) care should be taken when working on those with an intrauterine contraceptive device in situ, as the downwards movement could cause expulsion of the coil (and has been known to occur). Once familiar with locating the position of the zone for the cervix, the downwards movement should be omitted (see Fig. 3.3).

Fallopian tubes and pelvic lymphatics

The fallopian tubes join the ovaries to the uterus, therefore the zones are found as a line running across the top of each foot, similar to an ankle strap on a shoe. When learning, it is easier, first, to locate the ovary zone on the outer heel and the corresponding uterus point on the inner heel and then to identify the "ankle strap" line running across the top of the foot, below the ankle bones, which represents the fallopian tube. On either side of the tubes lie the zones for the pelvic lymphatics. During a treatment session, if it is appropriate to use the "caterpillar crawling" movement specifically over the zones for the reproductive tract, it is important to work *from* the ovary *to* the uterus, i.e. from the outer aspect of the foot to the inner aspect, in the direction of the movement of the hair-like cilia within the tubes. Generally, also, the practitioner would work the whole reproductive tract, from the ovary and across the fallopian tube to the uterus zones (Figs 3.2, 3.3).

Vagina and perineum

Having identified the zones for the uterine cavity and, below that, the cervix, the vaginal zone can be located. This is a continuation of the imaginary line dissecting the right angle of the inner heel, working towards the apex of the 90° angle. The zone for the perineum is at the very distal edge of the heel, an area which can often be very tender in the early puerperium if the mother has had an episiotomy or severe perineal laceration which has been sutured (Figs 3.2, 3.3). It may also appear very dark red in the days immediately following delivery.

The breasts and axillary lymphatics

The mammary glands are also important in maternity-related RZT, but, unlike some zones for the reproductive organs, those for the breasts are more easily located. The breast zones occupy the first one-third of the dorsal surface of the foot, being the soft tissue ranging from the midline to the distal edge of the dorsum below the bases of the toes. During the menstrual cycle of the non-pregnant woman these areas of the feet may be tender and even become slightly swollen ("puffy") in the pre-menstrual phase if the woman suffers breast tenderness. Similarly, in early pregnancy the upper dorsal surface can be uncomfortable when pressed firmly, whilst in the early puerperium it will be tender, swollen and sometimes reddish in colour until lactation becomes established. The nipple zone can be located by dividing the whole zone into four; the point at which all four quadrants meet is the usual location of the nipple zone. This may or may not be tender during pregnancy but will certainly inflict a sharp stinging pain when pressed firmly if the mother has sore nipples in the puerperium. A segmental area of acute tenderness in one of the breast zones during the puerperium may indicate a developing abscess and can be a useful diagnostic aid.

Unfortunately, in RZT, the breast zone is partly overlaid by the zone for the hand and forearm; therefore, it is necessary to become skilled at differentiating the depth of pressure required to work on either the hand or the breast. The expectant mother with carpal tunnel syndrome will have a precisely located point on the upper dorsum, which corresponds to her hand

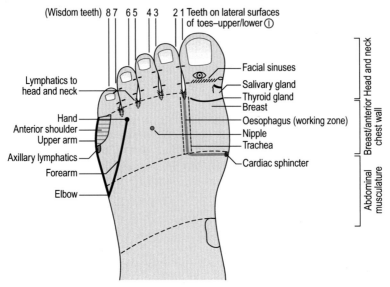

(Wisdom teeth) 8 7 6 5 4 3 2 1 Teeth on lateral surfaces
of toes–upper/lower ⓘ

Lymphatics to head and neck

Hand
Anterior shoulder
Upper arm

Axillary lymphatics

Forearm

Elbow

Facial sinuses
Salivary gland
Thyroid gland
Breast
Oesophagus (working zone)
Nipple
Trachea

Cardiac sphincter

Breast/anterior Head and neck chest wall

Abdominal musculature

Fig. 3.4   Reflex zones on dorsum of foot (left)

zone, whereas the tenderness elicited from the breast zone will be felt only when a deeper pressure is used (Figs 3.3, 3.4). The axillary lymphatics, which may need to be treated in newly delivered mothers with breast engorgement, are found on the distal edge of the foot below the zone for the scapula on the plantar surface and mirrored on the dorsal surface (Figs 3.1, 3.4).

DIAGNOSTIC POTENTIAL OF THE REFLEX ZONES FOR THE REPRODUCTIVE ORGANS

Although most textbooks state that reflexology should not be used to diagnose conditions, it is certainly possible to elicit from the feet a number of changes which appear to indicate altered physiology, even if only at a systematic level (Raz et al 2003). However, a small study by White et al (2000) identified discrepancies between the various reflexology charts or maps, while Baerheim et al (1998) found that there was a tendency of reflexologists to "over-diagnose", i.e. to "discover" pathology where none appeared to exist. Conversely, an earlier investigation by Omura (1994), in which an attempt was made to chart the feet using Bi-Digital O-Ring test resonance, claimed to correlate several assumed foot reflex zones with the organs that they are meant to represent.

There is, however, an increasing interest in this diagnostic potential. This has evolved from the anecdotal practice of "reading the feet", originated by Ingham and Byers (1992) and the esoteric, non-academic claims that the feet inform the practitioner of personality traits and psycho-emotional aspects of the whole (Stormer 2007), to an emerging evidence base supporting the use of reflex zones in the identification of changing physiology and impending pathology. This author has a particular interest in the diagnostic potential of reflexology, and has used it on numerous occasions to identify current, previous or impending conditions in pregnant and childbearing women.

CASE STUDY I   IDENTIFICATION OF PRE-ECLAMPSIA

Lesley, a gravida 4, para 3 at 33 weeks' gestation, was referred to the complementary therapy (CT) midwife's clinic with moderate hypertension, having been seen the day before, at home, by her community midwife, who thought that Lesley would benefit from some relaxation therapy. Following an initial consultation, Lesley readily agreed to try reflex zone therapy (RZT). Nothing untoward was revealed during the visual examination and the CT midwife started the palpatory stage of the treatment. However, on palpation of the second and third toes on each foot, the reflex zones for the eyes, Lesley reported extremely sharp tenderness. In a flash of inspiration, the CT midwife asked Lesley how long she had experienced flashing lights in front of her eyes, at which point Lesley burst into tears. It transpired that she had suffered visual disturbances for about a day and a half, but although the community midwife had asked her about this the day before, Lesley had lied about it because she did not want to be admitted to hospital, leaving her three children, all of whom were under 5, at home. The CT midwife took Lesley's blood pressure (BP), which was abnormally high at 170/100, although there were no other visual signs, and arranged to transfer her to the delivery suite for further investigations. Lesley's BP failed to respond to treatment and increased further over the next few hours. She was advised that it was best if the baby was delivered and later that evening she gave birth to a baby boy, by Caesarean section.

CASE STUDY 2   ASSISTING THE OBSTETRICIAN WITH A DIAGNOSIS

Mo was a 28-year-old gravid 3, para 2 who had been admitted 3 days ago to the antenatal ward, at 34 weeks' gestation, with unexplained severe abdominal pain, for which she was having a variety of investigations. She had previously had two Caesarean sections and an appendicectomy, and the senior registrar believed that her pain might be due to adhesions. However, the consultant was not so sure that Mo's pain was genuine because she spent a great deal of the day either outside the front doors of the maternity unit, smoking, or on her bed with the curtains drawn round, entertaining visitors and drinking alcohol. Despite this, she seemed to be awake through most of the night crying and when the day shift midwives came on duty she would be inconsolable with pain. The consultant was very supportive of the complementary therapies (CT) midwife and asked her to perform reflex zone therapy (RZT) in an attempt to offer a different perspective on Mo's diagnosis. The CT midwife invited Mo to have reflexology for relaxation and proceeded to perform a full treatment, which Mo enjoyed. However, whilst working over the reflex zone for the left kidney, Mo reported a sharp pain, and the CT midwife felt some irregularities in the zone, suggesting a possible renal condition. She reported back to the consultant, who ordered an intravenous urogram which revealed previously undiagnosed renal calculi, for which treatment was then instigated.

One aspect of diagnosis which appears, in the experience of this author, to be approximately 70% accurate, is the possibility of predicting stages of the menstrual cycle in non-pregnant women. Also, of specific relevance to maternity care is the information which can be gleaned from palpation of the pituitary gland reflex zones towards the end of pregnancy and which may assist in the prediction of labour, as well as other possible diagnostic tools related to the progress of labour (see Chapter 5).

Determining stages of the menstrual cycle

In the majority of women of reproductive age the zones for the pituitary gland will feel tender when thumb pressure is applied by the practitioner, a tenderness which varies according to the hormonal state of the individual. However, this is not an exact estimation but more of a "guesstimate" and, although this author has conducted a pilot study, no formal research has yet been completed. Factors such as an irregular cycle, the peri-menopausal phase and the use of hormones such as the contraceptive pill, a Mirena™ coil or hormone replacement therapy will obviously render this assessment unreliable.

The suggested routine to facilitate this prediction is shown in Box 3.1.

Box 3.1   Determining stages of the menstrual cycle

1. Determine whether the woman is in the follicular or luteal phase of her menstrual cycle:
   Experiential evidence appears to suggest that the pituitary zone on the right foot is tender throughout the menstrual cycle, whereas that on the left foot becomes increasingly more tender as the woman progresses from mid-cycle to menstruation (see also Tiran & Chummun 2005). Thus, by questioning the woman about the degrees of tenderness between the pituitary points on the two feet, it is possible to assess whether she is in the first part of her cycle (the follicular phase from menstruation to ovulation), or the latter 14 days (the luteal phase from ovulation to menstruation). In the follicular phase, the woman's right pituitary zone will be more tender, whereas in the luteal phase the left zone will be more uncomfortable. (A "tip" to remembering this system is to think "left = luteal/latter" part of the cycle).

2. Determine the active ovary for the current cycle:
   Gentle palpation of the two zones for the ovaries will also elicit tenderness, which is usually more dominant on one foot. As mentioned above, this appears to indicate the active ovary for the current cycle – i.e. the ovary on which the Graafian follicle is developing or the corpus luteum is declining. A formal research study would need to confirm this with vaginal ultrasound scans.

3. Determine the day of the cycle:
   Finally, palpating the zone for the fallopian tube on the side of the active ovary appears to suggest not only the anatomical reflex zone but also to correspond to a period of approximately 14 days in women with an average cycle. This is consistent with the two phases of the menstrual cycle (whilst remembering that the first – follicular – phase may be longer or shorter than 14 days, dependent on the length

of the woman's cycle). By asking the woman to indicate where – precisely – she feels most tenderness as the practitioner palpates across the fallopian tube zone, an estimate of the number of days in the relevant phase of the menstrual cycle can be made. There may be several points of tenderness along this area, so it is important to define which is most tender. For example, the woman may report most tenderness at the mid-point of the fallopian tube zone, on the apex of the "sandal strap" area. This would suggest that she is either 7 days or 21 days through her menstrual cycle, depending on whether she is in the follicular or luteal phase, as defined by the pituitary zone palpation. Degrees of tenderness can be identified and compared by using a scale of 1–10, with 1 being no tenderness and 10 equalling extreme tenderness.

HEAD AND NECK

The two big toes represent the head and neck in miniature, whilst the other toes correspond to the eyes and ears. Bearing in mind that the dorsal surface relates to the front of the body, the dorsal surfaces of the two big toes offer a map of the face, while the plantar surfaces represent the back of the head. The frontal, parietal, occipital, temporal and mandibular bones can, therefore, also be identified. The nails are not palpated during treatment in RZT but facilitate location of the orbital ridge; above the nail is the zone for the forehead. However, palpation of the nails can sometimes be uncomfortable suggesting that the reflex zones for the forehead lie also underneath the nails. Soft tissues of the head include the mouth, salivary glands, tonsils and thyroid gland on the dorsum and the Eustachian tube at the base of the plantar surface. Reflex zones for the facial musculature and nerve supply extend over the entire surface of all ten toes. The zones for the lymphatic system of the head and neck are located in the webbing between the toes, on both the dorsal and plantar surfaces; lymphatic drainage in this area can be facilitated by sweeping the webbing with a slight pinching movement of the thumb and forefinger (Figs 3.1, 3.4). This technique is usually included in the general relaxation treatment but is also particularly useful when treating headaches.

The second and third toes relate to the eye, with the second representing the inner, medial aspect of each eye and the third the distal aspect; the lacrimal duct is a tiny line extending medially from the lower edge of each inner eye zone. The dorsal surface of these two toes actually corresponds to the cornea, whereas the plantar surface relates to the retina, since this is anatomically situated behind the cornea. The fourth and fifth toes relate to the ears, with the fifth being the outer ear and the fourth being the middle and inner ear. The bony tips of toes 2 to 5 also represent the vault of the skull. It is worth noting that women with worsening pre-eclampsia who are beginning to develop symptoms may feel tenderness in the eye reflex zones if they are experiencing visual disturbances related to oedema around the optic nerve.

The teeth zones are located on the medial and distal sides of the toes, starting with tooth number 1 on the distal side of the big toe and tooth number 8, the wisdom tooth, on the medial aspect of toe 5. Upper teeth are above the interphalangeal joint of each toe, and the lower teeth are below this line. It may be possible to elicit a response from the mother when pressing on the zone corresponding to any tooth which needs a filling or which has had dental work performed on it, even many years previously. However, pregnant women frequently report tenderness in all the teeth zones, on both feet; this is more likely to reflect sore and bleeding gums or gingivitis, which is a common condition in pregnancy due to the increased blood supply to the area (Fig. 3.4).

Lett (2000:205–211) explores the concept that the reflex zones for the teeth are an energy field in their own right, in the same way as the feet, hands and back. This is based on the work of the early 20th century RZT authorities, including Fitzgerald, Bowers and Starr White and further investigations in the 1980s by German acupuncturists, who found relationships between individual teeth and distal organs and structures of the body. It is not, however, the intention of this book to consider this advanced theory in depth at this juncture, and readers are referred to the discussion and references in Lett (2000; Chapter 11).

MUSCULOSKELETAL SYSTEM

The system of RZT used by this author has been termed *"Structural reflex zone therapy"* as it focuses particularly on misalignments in the musculoskeletal system, in a similar way to osteopathy, but uses the reflex zones of the feet to attempt to correct these deviations (see Chapter 1). It will be seen in Chapters 4–6 that a comprehensive knowledge of the zones for the various components of the musculoskeletal system can aid practice and the effectiveness of treatment, not only during pregnancy and the puerperium, but also during labour. Again, readers familiar with generic reflexology may be challenged by the variations in some of the zones, which this author feels differ slightly, even from those zones identified by Marquardt (2000:40) and Lett (2000:148–149).

Spine

It is easiest to remember that, on the feet, soft tissue reflects soft tissue and organs, whilst the bony parts of the feet correspond to the bony parts of the body. Thus the spine runs down the medial aspect of both feet, from the inner tip of the big toe and along the bony inner edge of the foot towards the heel. When working the spine area, even during a relaxation treatment, the "caterpillar crawling" movement should proceed along the reflex zone for the whole spine, from the big toe to the heel – from the cervical vertebrae to the coccyx. This encourages normalisation and a return to, or maintenance of, homeostasis within the spinal vertebrae and associated muscles and nerves. The procedure is then repeated, enabling more precise location and treatment of any specific vertebral zones. Some reflexology schools teach practitioners to return along the spine zone from coccyx to cervical vertebrae, but there is no apparent physiological justification for this and no other authority has been able to offer an acceptable reason for doing so (personal communications with reflexology teachers). The decisions regarding the precise nature of practice over the spine reflex zones are, therefore, a matter for individual rationalisation.

It is essential in structural RZT that practitioners are able to distinguish between the different sections of the spine; with experience, it should be possible to identify individual vertebrae. The seven cervical vertebrae, within the neck, run from the tip of the big toe to its base. The twelve thoracic vertebrae run from the base of the big toe to the peak of the arch of the foot. The five lumbar vertebrae run from this junction to the end of the arch, finishing just in front of the zone for the bladder. In the opinion of this author, the zones for the sacral and coccygeal vertebrae pass *behind* the bladder zone, not across it as so many practitioners believe, with the demarcation between sacral and coccygeal vertebrae being at the mid-point as the spine zone passes behind the bladder (see Fig. 3.3). This is perhaps justifiable as it more naturally follows the bony edge of the inner foot and mirrors the curve of the sacro-coccygeal section of the pelvic basin. Also, returning to the notion of "working" or "indirect" zones, locating the lower spine zones as they are here, appears to produce better results than the traditional position.

It is possible, in the spine zones, to identify lesions such as displaced intervertebral discs, or the presence of surgically implanted metal supports, which will be felt as a nodular area or a rigid, hard line respectively. Of course it is not usually possible to identify precisely what these nodules or hardness represent unless the mother has given a relevant history. Many women with pre-existing back problems, including muscular strain and more pathological conditions, will, during pregnancy, report tenderness in the feet in the zones corresponding to the precise location of the original discomfort as well as in the reflex zones related to the location of current symptoms.

The shoulder girdle, upper limbs, ribs and abdominal muscles

The reflex zone for the scapula is one of the easiest to locate, being the broad area of bone on the plantar surface of each foot at the top of the distal metatarsal, nearest the junction with the toes. The zone for the trapezius muscle, on the plantar surface, runs from the junction between toes 1 and 2, across the top of the ball of the foot, below toes 2, 3 and 4 (just below the Eustachian tube zone), and merges into the scapula at its medial edge. The upper arm zone is the bony distal edge of the foot, running from the scapula to the basal edge of the fifth metatarsal, the point at which the elbow zone is located. On the dorsum, a line running over the junctions of the first, second and third phalanges with the corresponding metatarsal bones, gives us the zone for the clavicle. In RZT, as opposed to some forms of generic reflexology, the forearms and hands are assumed to be positioned across the chest (but not crossed over). It is easier to locate the hand zone first, by palpating the dorsum just below toe 4, where a small dip will be felt. Once the hand zone has been identified the forearm zone is a straight line between the elbow and the hand zones (Figs 3.1, 3.4, 3.5).

The rib cage zone is the bony metatarsal section of the dorsal surface, across the whole upper one third of the foot, and is overlaid first by the breast and then by the forearm and hand (see above). The sternum is on the medial dorsal edge of the foot over the metatarsal bones and the xiphisternum is the point at which the metatarsal meets the cuneiform bone.

The lower two-thirds of the dorsum, stretching as far as the fallopian tube/pelvic lymphatic zones, correspond to the zone for the abdominal musculature. In women with lax abdominal muscles this area may feel, on palpation,

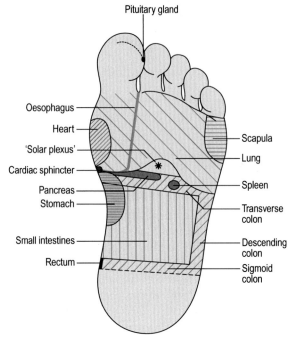

Fig. 3.5   Reflex zones on sole (left)

that it lacks tension. It may be possible to observe an apparent longitudinal division in mothers with divarification of the rectus sheath muscles, although this tends to be in the middle of *each* foot, in zone 3, rather than in the logical midline of the body in zone 1. If the woman has previously had abdominal surgery, she may report tenderness on palpation, and a shadowy line may be seen on the dorsal surface of the foot in the area relating to the site of abdominal scarring. Interestingly, however, these too are usually located in zone 3 on both feet as opposed to zone 1.

The bony pelvis

The bony pelvis is obviously of significance in maternity RZT, the lateral boundaries being the inner and outer ankle bones. The outer ankle bone on each foot represents the zone for the hip, while the inner ankle bones correspond to the symphysis pubis. In women experiencing, or beginning to develop, symphysis pubis discomfort or diastasis, the lower 180° of the inner ankle bone may take on a brownish or bruised-looking discolouration, which on palpation will feel tender to touch; often this is unilateral and may be accompanied by sciatica on the same side of the body.

The zone for the musculature of the pelvis is found on the plantar surface of the heels. It is fascinating to observe that, in pregnant women, the skin in this area of the heels frequently becomes excessively dry as pregnancy progresses, to the extent of becoming hard, scaly and flaking. This may simply be due to the altered centre of gravity which occurs with increased weight and more pronounced lumbar lordosis, the mother's weight being directed backwards as she places her feet on the ground with each step. However, since the pelvic musculature and ligaments are constantly being stretched during the antenatal period, often causing groin pain, it may be that this alteration in skin texture also reflects compromised homeostasis in the pelvic region.

Further landmarks can be found which are fundamental to treatment during pregnancy and labour. The sacroiliac joint, through which the sciatic nerve passes, is located behind the outer ankle bone, at an angle of approximately 35° from the midline; it is found by tucking the finger tip behind and under the bone, where a small indentation can be felt. From this point, the zone for the sciatic nerve runs in a perpendicular line parallel to the posterior aspect of the leg. However, it is vital to distinguish the sacroiliac joint reflex zone from that of the Bladder 60 acupuncture point, as stimulation of the latter may initiate contractions and is contraindicated until term. Whilst this may be a useful acupressure point to use immediately before and during labour, it would be inappropriate to stimulate this as a result of mistaking it for the sacroiliac reflex zone (see Figs 3.2, 3.3 and Chapter 5).

The lower limbs

It is interesting that there are no real zones for the lower limbs below those for the knees. Any condition of the legs below the knees would be treated with specific reflex zone techniques applied either to the opposite leg, in a mirror image of the relevant area, or on the hands.

The basic reflex zone charts, used by both Marquardt (2000:7) and Lett (2000:18), give the appearance of a person sitting upright with the legs stretched out in front. The thigh zone, therefore, logically extends from the outer ankle bone (the hip zone) for about three finger-breadths perpendicularly up the back of the leg, following the line of the lower fibula (alongside that for the sciatic nerve) and ending at a point which reflects the direct reflex zone for the knee. In her earlier publication, Marquardt (1983:46) queries the location for the knee reflex zone, but suggests another, at a point on the lateral rim of the heel, directly inferior to the outer malleolus. She suggests that, logically, this should relate to the reflex zone for part of the (bony) pelvic region, but comments that, the knees can be treated at this point as it is also a reflex zone for the nerves which supply the legs. However, there appears to be another indirect zone for the knee which is more easily located, and which more readily reveals changes in the knees during pregnancy. This is found, somewhat illogically, on the dorsum, in front of the hip zone, suggesting perhaps that, instead of sitting with the legs in front, the reflex zone map reflects a person crouching on their knees (Fig. 3.2). Lett's original text (1983:119) concurs with this suggestion, but her subsequent text (2000:124) appears to refute it. Certainly, in pregnancy, as maternal weight increases, there is considerable pressure placed on the knee joints, to the extent that they may abduct slightly in the third trimester, the joints and ligaments being unduly stressed. Many women complain of pain or discomfort in their knees and the feet often reveal the extent of this problem, with the apparently indirect (working) zones for the knees becoming oedematous, deep bluish in colour and tender to touch.

LYMPHATIC SYSTEM

The lymphatic system consists of various lymph glands, the thymus, spleen, tonsils and appendix. Whilst most of the organs do not usually have a direct relevance to pregnancy RZT, it is necessary to be aware of their location as any irregularities found either on inspection or palpation may alert the practitioner to underlying variations in physiology or previous, current or impending pathology. As mentioned above, the reflex zones for the head and neck lymphatics are located in the webbing between each of the toes. The axillary lymphatic zones are found at the base of the shoulder joint zones where a slight indentation is felt, and the zones for the pelvic/groin lymphatics are easily located across the dorsal surface of each foot, in a line either side of the fallopian tubes, corresponding to the ankle strap of a sandal. The entire plantar, medial and distal aspects of the heel relate to the reflex zones for the pelvis, which will be worked during any relaxation treatment.

The zone for the *spleen* is on the left foot only (the same zone on the right foot is the reflex zone for the gallbladder). With the plantar surface of the foot clearly visible and the big toe perpendicular to the ceiling, draw an imaginary line down from the fourth toe to a point just below the diaphragm, slightly distal to the relaxation point ("solar plexus"). The spleen is a vascular organ of self-defence, producing antibodies and white blood corpuscles and metabolising old red corpuscles, and the reflex zone may, therefore, be tender to touch in the presence of upper abdominal or haematological conditions, allergies and cardiac pathology. Occasionally, the spleen is lost, either through disease or injury, and its functions are then taken over by other organs, such as the liver, lymph nodes and bone marrow. However, the original reflex zone for the spleen will remain tender to direct touch and a small indentation may be felt on palpation (Fig. 3.5).

The zones for the *tonsils* are situated on the distal edge at the base of the big toes at a precise point on the lower outer edge in close proximity to the webbing that constitutes the lymphatic zones. If the mother develops an upper respiratory tract infection she will experience a sharp tenderness in this zone; if she has had a tonsillectomy, a bruised sensation will occur on palpation of the zone. This tenderness can be quite intense even when the tonsils have been removed, which differs from the mild bruised sensation usually experienced on palpation of zones relating to other organs that have been surgically removed. The *thymus gland* is involved in regulating the immune system through the production of T cells. It is located on the medial edge of the first metatarsal on the dorsal surface of the big toes, approximately in line with the lower end of the oesophagus. The *vermiform appendix* is located in the right iliac fossa, the reflex zone, therefore, being found on the right foot only, on the plantar surface on the edge of the calcaneum and on the medial edge of the beginning of the reflex zone for the ascending colon (Fig. 3.1). In women who have had their appendix removed there may be tenderness on palpation and a noticeable dip at this point.

RENAL TRACT

During pregnancy the renal tract is compromised by hormonal and structural changes, including increased frequency of micturition and an altered glomerular filtration rate; there is also an increased possibility of urinary tract infection due to stasis of urine in the ureters as a result of progesterone relaxation and dilatation of the ureteric lumen. Therefore, it is *essential* that the zones for the renal tract are only worked *from* the zones for the kidney, *down* the ureter and *towards* the bladder; treatment should *never* be in the reverse direction, especially during pregnancy, as this could theoretically transfer bladder pathogens to the kidneys, potentially leading to pyelonephritis. This may challenge many reflexologists who are taught to work in both directions along the renal tract but who are unable to justify this practice and who, when treating pregnant clients, fail to take into account the delicate balance of the urinary system in the antenatal period.

Kidneys

The kidney zone is located on the plantar surface of each foot in line with zone 2 and below the line for the diaphragm (Fig. 3.1, applicable to both feet). These zones may be tender when palpated during pregnancy, simply because renal function (glomerular filtration) is altered at this time. However, if one kidney zone is significantly more tender than the other, it may lead the practitioner to suspect that a urinary tract infection is developing even before the mother experiences any symptoms, such as dysuria or excessive frequency of micturition. The mother should be asked to produce a midstream urine specimen for laboratory analysis to exclude infection or to determine the most appropriate antibiotic treatment and no further RZT should be performed directly on these zones until the signs and symptoms have subsided. Untreated bladder infection can track upwards and develop into pyelonephritis, with a grave risk to the fetus as well as the mother and the risk of preterm labour.

Care should also be taken when working over the zones for the kidneys if there is any reason to suspect renal calculi; theoretically, over-stimulation could move a kidney stone from a largish duct to one which is much smaller, which would then lead to considerable acute pain.

Ureters and bladder

The zone for the ureter, on each foot, is a straight line between the kidney and the bladder zones. Whilst it is important to work down the ureter zone before working the bladder zone, in practice it is easier, when learning, to locate the bladder zone first. The bladder is an organ in the midline of the body, thus the two halves of the bladder zone are located in zone 1, on the medial aspect of each foot. In many people this point is very noticeable, as a slightly bulbous area in front of the heel. However, when the zone is not visibly identifiable the practitioner should look for the point at which the heel starts to rise into the arch of the foot, then take a perpendicular line up towards the inner ankle bone (see Figs 3.1, 3.3, 3.5). The bladder zone may be tender to touch in the presence of an infection. Postnatally, it may also be tender if there has been trauma during labour or delivery, such as a prolonged first stage with bladder compression or a difficult forceps delivery. Contrary to popular belief, it does not necessarily enlarge when the bladder is full, neither does it reduce in size once the bladder is emptied!

GASTROINTESTINAL TRACT

Mouth, salivary glands and oesophagus

The mouth zone is situated on the dorsal surface of the big toe, with half being in the midline of each foot; those for the salivary glands emerge from the distal edge of the two halves of the mouth zone (Fig. 3.4). It is necessary to develop sufficiently precise clinical skills to identify these areas as many pregnant women experience hypersalivation (ptyalism), either as a component of gestational sickness or in isolation.

The oesophagus is represented on both the dorsal and plantar surfaces of the feet, but this is another example of a zone being placed in an area of the feet that does not logically comply with gross anatomical positioning. Since the oesophagus is central to the body, it should be located in zone 1. However, tradition and practice place it between zones 1 and 2, i.e. between the big toe and toe 2. Furthermore, its anatomical relationship with the trachea suggests that the zones for the trachea and bronchi should be on the dorsum and that for the oesophagus on the plantar surface. Lett (1983:49; 2000:159) and Marquardt (2000:67–68) both site the oesophagus zones on the two surfaces of the feet, although their points of insertion commence, as one might expect, in the mouth zones on the dorsum. They also suggest that these zones are superimposed on those for the trachea, again on both surfaces of the feet (Lett 2000:155; Marquardt 2000:65). In practice, this author feels that the true zone for the oesophagus is on the plantar surface but the working – or indirect – zone is on the dorsal surface, with the zones for the trachea running either side (Figs 3.1, 3.4, 3.5). Although there is no anatomical logic to this, clinical practice has shown that women suffering heartburn and indigestion during pregnancy also have tenderness in this area of the feet, and effective resolution can be achieved by sedating the relevant points, dependent on the exact location of the symptoms.

Cardiac sphincter and stomach

The stomach lies anatomically below the diaphragm, in a central position but displaced to the left. On the feet, the reflex zones are on the medial aspect of each foot, in zone 1, with a larger area for the zone on the left foot. The oesophagus naturally joins the stomach at the cardiac sphincter, which is on the medial aspect as a very precise point below the line for the diaphragm, and in front of the spine (towards the dorsal surface) (see Figs 3.1, 3.5). Although this location differs slightly from Lett (2000:160), in practice it is the most relevant point for treating indigestion and heartburn.

Intestines, rectum and anus

The ascending colon of the large intestines is on the distal aspect of the right foot, the transverse colon crosses from right to left in a horizontal line below the diaphragm and the descending colon runs down the distal aspect of the left foot, all on the plantar surfaces. The small intestines curl round in a clockwise direction inside the boundaries of the large intestines. When viewed on the plantar surface of the feet the whole of the intestines can be seen and would normally be worked by alternating from one foot to the other, commencing on the right foot. This is a reason quoted by many practitioners for starting any RZT treatment on the right foot, but is not necessary for a general relaxation session. In women who require specific stimulation of the gastrointestinal tract, as with constipation, the two feet can be uncovered and stimulating techniques used in a clockwise direction from the right to the left foot. Lett (2000:159) and Marquardt (2000:67/8) further differentiate the anatomical sections of the gastrointestinal tract (e.g. duodenum, ileocaecal valve, sigmoid colon, etc.), but this is not usually necessary in maternity RZT and has been omitted here.

The zone for the rectum is at the base of the descending colon, as the lower border of the large intestines returns to the midline, although Lett (2000) locates it on the medial aspect of the calcaneum. This is perhaps more logical, especially since the anal sphincter zone is found on the very top of the calcaneum – but on both the medial *and* the distal sides of the feet (in the area of the Achilles tendon) (see Figs 3.1, 3.2, 3.3, 3.5). There may be redness on one or both feet and on one or both sides of either foot in the event of developing haemorrhoids, and women with symptoms will also feel tenderness at these points. The discomfort will be dull and bruise-like if the mother had haemorrhoids in a previous pregnancy or they are just beginning to develop, but may be a sharp and acute pain if the haemorrhoids are prolapsed and bleeding.

ENDOCRINE SYSTEM

The pituitary gland, the reproductive organs and the breast (mammary gland) have already been discussed (see above). In men the reproductive organs correspond to those in the female – the ovaries/testes; fallopian tubes/inguinal canal and vas deferens; the uterus/prostate gland and scrotum; and the vagina/penis.

Thyroid gland

The zone for the thyroid gland is located on the dorsal surface at the base of the big toes, on the joints where the toes join the foot. In pregnancy these zones often become slightly tender due to increased thyroid activity, especially when the mother is suffering nausea and vomiting, when they also develop a brownish or greyish appearance, sometimes in a line which covers the whole width of the big toes. It is vital to be aware of the mother's relevant history, including the prescription of any thyroid medication, before attempting to "treat" the thyroid zone, since stimulation or sedation could upset the delicate physiological balance (see Fig. 3.4).

Adrenal glands

The adrenal glands are positioned superiorly to the kidneys, therefore it is essential to locate the kidney zones before doing any reflex treatment on the adrenals (see Renal tract, above). The only real indication for working specifically on the zones for the adrenal glands is to treat panic and acute anxiety by sedating the zones to suppress the output of adrenaline (epinephrine). This can be achieved by locating the kidney zones, then placing the thumb tips precisely over them. By bending the thumbs the tips will then dip over the kidney zones and into the adrenal areas; a brief pause of no more than 5 seconds at a time should be sufficient to lower the adrenaline to a more normal level. Sustained pressure on these points can lead to extreme dizziness and fainting, especially during pregnancy, and the points should only be used occasionally for acute stress and *not* for general relaxation (Fig. 3.1, applicable to both feet).

Pancreas

The pancreas zone lies on the plantar surface of both feet and is located below the diaphragm, above the stomach zone, predominating on the left foot. It is a thin sliver of a zone but can be easily over-stimulated if there is vigorous work over the reflex zone for the transverse colon (Fig. 3.5). This is particularly relevant in women with diabetes, although those who are insulin-dependent would not normally be eligible to receive RZT (see Chapter 2).

HEPATO-BILIARY SYSTEM

As the liver is anatomically situated on the right side of the body, the reflex zone for the liver appears only on the right foot. In gross anatomy the liver is the largest internal organ in the body, and in reflexology, this is also true. The liver zone is below the diaphragm line, extending from the distal edge of the foot, to halfway across the plantar surface, its medial edge being found in line with zone 3. In reality there is a natural wedge-shaped edge to the foot which naturally delineates the borders for the liver, the lower edge being the junction between the arch of the foot and the heel (Fig. 3.1).

However, the liver zone is overlain by the ascending colon and part of the small intestines, whilst the gall bladder zone is a precise point on the upper edge of the liver zone. This can make it difficult for the novice to differentiate the zones, but with experience varying pressures will facilitate appropriate treatment. The liver zone may feel tender to touch when there is a need within the body for detoxification, such as following the use of various drugs in labour. The hand zone for the liver is on the right hand, and is the fleshy area below the main crease across the palm, on the distal edge, in line with the little finger. Sometimes detoxification can be achieved more easily by working on the hands as this wedge-shaped area can be massaged by the mother using her left hand.

Gall bladder

The gall bladder is situated on the superior surface of the liver, therefore the reflex zone is found only on the right foot. With the plantar surface of the foot clearly visible and the big toe perpendicular to the ceiling, draw an imaginary line down from the fourth toe to a point just below the diaphragm, slightly distal to the relaxation point (see Fig. 3.1). (The spleen zone is located in exactly the same position on the left foot, see Fig. 3.5.) The gall bladder zone may feel tender when the mother has eaten a high-fat meal but this should not be taken as a sign of pathology, unless there is reason to suspect calculi or other problem. However, in the event of suspected or current gall stones, or a personal or family history of the condition, *no* direct work – stimulation or sedation – should be undertaken on this precise point, to avoid exacerbating the condition. Theoretically, if one takes the principle of RZT being able to "move things along tubes" (see Chapter 2), poor technique or over-exuberant working of the area may result in dislodging a gallstone from one duct into a smaller – and more painful – duct. The area will be treated indirectly as part of the overall assessment and relaxation treatment, and this is usually sufficient.

CARDIO-RESPIRATORY SYSTEM

Heart

The heart reflex zone is above the line for the diaphragm on the medial aspect of each foot, with a slightly larger zone on the left foot than on the right, as the heart is centrally located in the thoracic cavity but slightly displaced to the left. The heart zone is the soft tissue situated on the dorsal, medial and plantar surfaces of each foot at the junction of the phalange and metatarsal on the big toe; care should be taken not to confuse this with the lower end of the bone – which corresponds to the neck. Further sub-divisions are possible, the zones for the aortic arch and superior vena cava being above the heart zone and the descending aorta and inferior vena cava being below, but these have been omitted here (Figs 3.1, 3.5).

Lungs

The lung zones are situated on the plantar surface of the foot and are the "balls" of the feet (Figs 3.1, 3.5). "Caterpillar crawling" movements can be applied across this whole area during a relaxation treatment, or the balls of the feet can be held with the practitioner's palms firmly pressed against them. Gentle working of the zones for the lungs can aid relaxation and ease breathing, particularly when the mother is hyperventilating, as may occur during labour contractions.

When inspecting the lung zones, areas of hard skin may be seen, which are usually attributed to the pressure placed on the feet when walking, but which may also give an indication of abnormal alignment of the pelvis, especially if the distribution is irregular and uneven. The surface of the lung zones may be whitish in colour or vary from yellow to red. Yellowing skin may reflect some impairment of the respiratory system, and is particularly common in smokers, but can also suggest that the woman suffers from asthma or other chronic respiratory condition. When the skin is reddish it is more likely to relate to a recent or current infection or irritation in the respiratory tract, such as a cold, influenza or hay fever. Later in pregnancy, reddish skin may alert the practitioner to obstetric-related issues, such as shortness of breath from upwards pressure of the fetus against the diaphragm, which compresses the bases of the lungs. However, it is important to determine whether or not this is physiological or pathological, for example breathlessness resulting from severe anaemia requires different treatment from shortness of breath caused by the anatomical adaptations of pregnancy. Occasionally a broad indentation or whitish line is observed on the surface of the ball of the foot, between the first and second toes. This can also indicate respiratory compromise, but may instead reflect oesophageal problems, commonly (but not exclusively) being heartburn and indigestion in pregnant women (see Gastrointestinal tract, above).

Structural reflex zone therapy for pregnancy

4

CHAPTER CONTENTS

INTRODUCTION

Expectant mothers experience myriad physical symptoms and emotional upheavals as pregnancy progresses, and their needs vary according to the gestation. This chapter outlines suggested structural reflex zone therapy (RZT) treatments for a variety of physiological problems which occur in the antenatal period. The approach used here is intended to facilitate readers to relate specific RZT techniques to the aetiology and relevant physiology, from a musculoskeletal (or *structural*) perspective, and to consider how reflexology complements conventional medical and/or midwifery management. The conventional theories regarding physiology and management are included here only where it relates to structural RZT treatment and readers requiring a more in-depth knowledge of the conditions are referred to the lists of further reading and resources. Practitioners should also bear in mind that, whilst the suggestions given for treatment may be suitable in many cases, they can only be a general guide and it is important to consider the specific needs of each individual mother. Indeed, there is no real formulaic "recipe" which can be given for treating a particular condition – because it is not the *condition* which is being treated, but the mother (and fetus) as a whole. Furthermore, mothers frequently complain of several symptoms occurring simultaneously; the skill and experience of the practitioner will enable him/her to determine whether to treat each symptom separately (although not in isolation) or whether to provide a complete holistic treatment which goes beyond the realms of a simple relaxation treatment. If there is any doubt about the justification for specific treatment, the mother should be given only a light relaxation treatment – or the practitioner should refrain from treating her at all.

> There is no pre-determined set of reflex zone therapy techniques for treating particular pregnancy conditions: practitioners need to consider the specific needs of each individual mother in order to treat her appropriately and holistically.

INFERTILITY AND PRECONCEPTION CARE

Infertility is not a condition encountered by many midwives, but numerous reflexologists are approached by women desperate to conceive (Coulson & Jenkins 2005, Stankiewicz et al 2007). There is a contemporary belief, amongst both the general public and inexperienced reflexologists, that "reflexology *treats* infertility", but this is not the case and therapists place themselves in an invidious professional position by making unfounded and sometimes blatantly untrue claims which do nothing to enhance the credibility of the profession as a whole – and therapists should be cautious of giving false hope to desperate people. There is no research evidence to demonstrate the success rates of reflexology for couples with infertility, although there are several case studies in both the popular and professional press (Kissinger & Kaczmarek 2006). It is interesting to note that only those who successfully conceive appear to find the experience of receiving reflexology for infertility empowering (Porter & Bhattacharya 2008). Sub-fertility is a complex condition which can affect either or both partners and specific treatment (conventional as well as complementary) can only be given once the cause has been identified. Couples who have been attempting to become pregnant after actively having regular unprotected sexual intercourse for at least 2 years (1 year in women over 35) are considered to have problems with fertility.

Structural physiology and aetiology

Causes of infertility may be structural, hormonal, psycho-social or educational, or they may be related to lifestyle and/or environmental factors; although about 25% of cases occur without any clear reason being found. In the woman, failure to ovulate may be triggered by excessive weight loss or gain, or conditions such as polycystic ovary syndrome. In those who ovulate, the ovum may be unable to reach the sperm due to blocked fallopian tubes following salpingitis or in the presence of endometriosis, or the cervical mucus may be hostile to the partner's semen, preventing conception. The commonest cause in men is sperm abnormalities, such as inadequate numbers of healthy sperm, or the presence of antisperm antibodies in the blood; testicular problems also contribute to the problem. Poor diet, smoking, alcohol and drug use (prescribed or recreational), as well as stressful lifestyles and occupations may cause sub-fertility or exacerbate the effects of other factors in both partners. Timing of sex may be inappropriate (either too little or too much, or not coinciding with ovulation), and occasionally lack of knowledge, or embarrassment, may mean that the relationship has not been consummated.

From a structural perspective, it is useful to explore the couple's previous medical histories in detail. Enquiries may reveal old injuries or accidents which could contribute to misalignment of the muscusloskeletal system, placing stress and tension on the organs of the reproductive tract or the endocrine system. If there has been any potential incident or disease in the past which may have a bearing on the current problem, alignment of the iliac crests (hips) should be measured and the therapist should take into account any other visible signs of misalignment such as walking with a limp or irregular positioning of clothing on the two sides of the body. Examples include: torticollis of the neck or a previous whiplash injury resulting in tension on the cervical vertebrae, which could interfere with the output of hormones from the pituitary gland, affecting ovulation and the menstrual cycle; or a fractured leg from an accident, which may cause persistent compensatory movements when walking, resulting in misalignment of the fallopian tubes. This creates tension due to over-stretching on one side, with stress on the ovary interfering with ovulation, whilst on the other side there is slackness of the tube and consequent poor transit of any ovum which is relased. In men, similar injuries may interefere with testosterone or sperm production or the transit of semen along the vas deferens.

Abnormal alignment of the bony pelvis, either congenitally or due to trauma or habitual positioning, may interfere with the alignment of the reproductive ligaments, causing problems such as a retroverted uterus. This puts additional strain on neighbouring organs, noticeably the sensitive fallopian tubes, within which any local disturbance may affect the peristaltic waves and interfere with transit of the ovum. In women with endometriosis, adhesions may create tensions which affect peristaltic movement of the uterus and fallopian tubes, and may cause torsion or spasm of the ovaries. Stress on the lower uterus blocks the cervical valve, causing neural or circulatory irritation which impedes the progress of the ascending sperm or the fertilised ovum. In men, the biomechanics of the hips, pelvic joints and lower back, the functioning of the pelvic floor musculature and the generalised circulation and nerve supply within the trunk and pelvis may contribute to subfertility, as may mechanical problems at the junction between the hypothalamus and the pituitary gland.

Relevant reflexology treatment

It is not the responsibility of the reflexologist to delve into all the possible causes of infertility and then to attempt to give advice or treatment that is outside the sphere of his/her knowledge and training; this would be unhelpful and unethical. In many couples, lifestyle factors undoubtedly contribute to sub-fertility, the reflexologist should not attempt to offer advice on aspects such as nutrition unless she is adequately qualified to do so. If reflexology is thought to be useful, it is ideal if both the woman and the man can be treated, not least to reduce their anxieties about the situation; this may also give an indication about who is in need of more specific therapy, if appropriate. It may also be possible to teach them to perform reflexology on each other, which may help to overcome some of the psycho-emotional issues which often accompany this problem. The therapist should also try not to feel too pressurised to succeed, as this can be transmitted to the client(s) and be counter-productive.

RZT treatment should focus primarily on relaxation in order to aid and restore homeostasis and to reduce the impact of excessive levels of stress hormones, which in itself can contribute to a failure to conceive (Cwikel et al 2004). RZT is thought to have positive effects on the immune system and, although specific reflexology research does not adequately support this (Lee 2006, McVicar et al 2007), investigations related to general touch and to massage demonstrate reduced cortisol levels following treatment (Garner et al 2008, Hernandez-Reif et al 2004), indicating a systemic de-stressing effect. Treatment may also be useful for relieving symptoms of related conditions, such as irritable bowel syndrome, premenstrual tension or other problems which may exacerbate, or be exacerbated by, stress. The woman may need to be treated over several menstrual cycles. The general relaxation reflexology treatment can then be followed by any RZT techniques aimed at treating the cause, if identified either from the practitioner's own assessment or from conventional medical investigations and if it is appropriate to do so.

> Reflexology does not "treat infertility" and there is no known reflex zone therapy technique which will "cure" this multifactorial problem. At best, reflexologists can provide treatment for women and their partners who are having difficulty in conceiving, and hope that the relaxation and harmonising effects help to restore homeostasis.

If the cause of female infertility has been found to be anovulation, perhaps due to a deficiency of pituitary hormones, reflexology may theoretically aid stimulation or rebalancing of the pituitary gland and facilitate maturation of the Graafian follicle, leading to ovulation in some, but not all, women. Stimulation of the pituitary gland reflex zone may be helpful in the event of non-ovulatory menstrual bleeds, although Holt et al (2008) found no statistically significant success rates either in inducing ovulation or in conception rates amongst women who received reflexology, compared to those who received sham reflexology/foot massage.

Stimulation of the foot zones for the ovaries should not be undertaken without justification and certainly not until polycystic ovary syndrome has been eliminated from the possible causes, as this may, theoretically, exacerbate the pathological effects. Any work on the reflex zones for the fallopian tubes must *always* be performed in the direction in which the cilia waft the ovum – from the ovary to the uterus zones. It is not usually appropriate to undertake any stimulating or sedating techniques on the uterine reflex zones unless there is specific uterine pathology – and in this case the practitioner will need first to determine which therapeutic technique is needed. For example, stimulation of the uterine zone in the presence of fibroids may precipitate haemorrhage or undue growth of the fibroids, causing pain, bleeding and anaemia.

Manipulative techniques (see Appendix 2) can be employed if there appears to be any structural misalignment, but care should be taken if the cause has not yet been identified. Specific manipulative treatment may be needed on the zones for the abdominal region, plus any areas of the spine indicating abnormal kyphosis or lordosis, which will also facilitate a return to homeostasis in the neighbouring muscles, nerves and lymphatics. Working on the reflex zones for the pelvic areas, in both women and men, including the bony pelvis, hips and lower back, as well as the ribs, may contribute to overall wellbeing in related reproductive and other organs, increasing circulation and possibly facilitating a toning of the muscles.

Reflexology will not, of course, treat anatomical deviations from the norm, including bicornuate uterus or, in men, abnormal testicular development such as undescended testes; nor will it relieve problems associated with abnormal pathology, including blocked fallopian tubes, hostile cervical mucus or anti-sperm antibodies. In these cases and in others where the cause is not yet known, the only purpose of reflexology is to relax the couple and to provide a "listening ear" for their anxieties. This does, however, require the practitioner to possess refined listening skills and to be sufficiently self-aware to appreciate his/her personal professional boundaries and to know when to stop listening and to refer on to a more appropriately trained counsellor.

Those who are referred by their family doctor for specialist infertility treatment may require particular care, both physiologically and psychologically, and RZT can be a beneficial complement to medical treatment. However, the practitioner should always communicate with the consultant gynaecologist to ensure that there is no adverse interaction between conventional and complementary treatments. It is the opinion of this author that *no* "hands on" treatment should be given, apart from very gentle stroking massage, during the times when the woman is taking ovulatory drugs (inhalation, patches or orally) or has just had fertilised embryos reimplanted in the uterus, in order to avoid any disruption to this delicate (and expensive) medical treatment, although RZT can be offered in the interim period and once a successful conception has become an established pregnancy (see also Chapter 2 for precautions).

STRESS, ANXIETY AND PANIC ATTACKS; TIREDNESS AND INSOMNIA

Structural physiology and aetiology

Women frequently experience feelings of anxiety during pregnancy; they may be worried about the baby or their own health, or the anticipation of the labour and birth may cause them to feel frightened. Personal, domestic, occupational, relationship or financial worries will increase the symptoms and the effects and may lead to pathological consequences. Some anxiety and fear is normal, but excessive negative emotions and long-term stress will interfere with materno-fetal health. Antenatal stress raises maternal cortisol levels which may lead to low fetal weight, intrapartum complications, impaired immune functioning in the neonate and poor cognitive development (Diego et al 2006, Ruiz & Avant 2005), which may even last for the duration of the offspring's lifespan (Sandman et al 2003). *Stress* increases the severity of relatively "minor" physiological symptoms such as nausea and vomiting or headaches in the first trimester and may lead to obstetric complications such as hypertension and pre-eclampsia (Sharma et al 2006). Chronic *anxiety* of more than 6 months' duration can have serious effects, including preterm labour and fetal loss (Bastard & Tiran 2006). *Panic attacks* are common in pregnancy and trigger physical reactions including a dry mouth, dizziness, palpitations or difficulty in breathing. Panic attacks may occur completely randomly with no apparent immediate cause, but can also be a component of depression (or a side effect of treatment for depression).

Tiredness is a normal aspect of early pregnancy as the mother's body adapts to and becomes accustomed to the raised hormone levels, and *insomnia* is common, particularly in the third trimester when sleep is interrupted by fetal movements, backache and other discomforts and frequency of micturition from bladder compression by the fetal head. However, unresolved tiredness can also affect the mother's ability to cope with normal physiological symptoms. Vivid dreams are common in late pregnancy, but tiredness and stress can turn these into nightmares which wake her, further affecting her sleep patterns and leading to the mother feeling unrefreshed on waking. This aggravates the situation and establishes a cycle of events from which it becomes difficult for the mother to extricate herself.

Whilst tiredness and the associated weariness can be worsened by pain and discomfort, the trio of emotional symptoms – stress, anxiety and tiredness – will also impact on the musculoskeletal sytem, affecting posture, exacerbating physiological backache and causing neck ache and headaches. Habitually poor posture from prolonged stress increases the kyphotic curvature of the thoracic spine, which constricts the anterior ribcage and compresses the upper stomach, thereby contributing to heartburn and indigestion. Restlessness – "tossing and turning" – at night can eventually lead to abnormal twisting of the spine as the mother attempts to get comfortable, and in severe cases may put excess strain on the sacroiliac joints and then indirectly on the whole bony pelvis, potentially increasing the risk of intrapartum problems such as occipitoposterior position of the fetus and prolonged labour. Compensatory posture during the day may also adversely affect alignment of the lower musculoskeletal system. This can lead to ligament strain, causing groin pain and symphysis pubis discomfort, and to pelvic constriction, especially from prolonged sitting, which affects circulation in the legs, causing oedema and varicosities.

It is, however, important to consider whether or not stress and anxiety, panic attacks, tiredness and insomnia constitute elements of a more pathological clinical depression, and to refer accordingly if this is suspected.

Relevant reflexology treatment

Any complementary therapy treatment aimed at aiding relaxation will be of help to the mother and fetus and it is in this context that reflexology has so much to offer. Psychologically, the treatment sessions provide the mother with some valuable "me time" and the opportunity to voice her concerns with someone whom she views as both a professional and, perhaps, as a friend. It is continually surprising how much the mother will "open up" during antenatal reflexology, a factor which is not seen in the same way amongst women who attend for massage or other complementary therapies or, indeed, for their normal antenatal appointments. This may be partly due to the mother being in an upright position, facilitating eye-to-eye contact, but may also result from the interaction required during the visual examination of the feet. Furthermore, when reflexology treatment is provided by midwives, particularly in an NHS setting, this may be seen as a luxury; the mother knows that she has a specified duration to her appointment, unlike the often rushed occasions for her routine antenatal examinations.

> Reflex zone therapy (RZT) provides holistic treatment, encompassing the psychological, emotional and physical aspects of health and wellbeing. Any RZT treatment for general psycho-emotional relaxation aims also to restore and maintain physiological homeostasis; and any specific treatments for physio-pathological conditions will work at a psychological level. Spiritual wellbeing is also facilitated through the overall experience of receiving a nurturing and individualised treatment and from the interaction between the client and the therapist.

Physiologically, the relaxation which can be achieved with RZT reduces the levels of circulating stress homones, such as adrenaline (epinephrine), noradrenaline (norepinephrine) and cortisol, lowering blood pressure and encouraging the release of endorphins and adequate levels of pregnancy hormones to assist in maintaining the health of the mother and fetus. Several research studies suggest that regular reflexology and other touch therapies in the last few weeks of pregnancy can also facilitate the progress and outcome of labour (Field et al 2008a, 2008b, McNeill et al 2006, Osborne 2008). This assists in regulating homeostasis by lowering stress hormones and increasing the output of oxytocin for labour. Treatment may comprise a general relaxation session of no longer than 30 minutes' duration (see Appendix 1), but it may also focus on the specific zones related to the exact symptoms and signs displayed by the mother.

Very gentle sedation of the relaxation point ("solar plexus" reflex zone) can precede and follow any other techniques, and be incorporated intermittently throughout the session, but any practitioner should be alert to the mother's response. Her fragile state can precipitate an emotional release during the session, such as bursting into tears or giggling uncontrollably. The relaxation point may be tender if the mother is very anxious and, in extreme cases, can be acutely painful, sometimes also appearing as a deep groove or dark greyish line down the centre of the foot, from the "solar plexus" point to the midpoint of the arch of the foot. If a mother has suffered prolonged (chronic) stress the entire surface of both feet may be tender, or she may report sharp sensations at a number of apparently unrelated points on the feet during the treatment. This does not necessarily imply that the mother has actual or impending pathology in each of the organs corresponding to the painful zones (although it may do), but is more likely to presage a chronic systemic effect. Similar, although usually less marked, responses are seen when the mother is very tired, perhaps because tiredness adversely affects the mother's coping abilities, generally making her more sensitive to painful stimuli. Often, of course, stress and tiredness occur simultaneously. However, the practitioner should work very gently over the feet and be sensitive to the maternal effects so that she can determine the time at which the treatment should end, as some women may not be able to tolerate a full 30 minute session.

Sweeping of the diaphragm zones can help to regulate uncoordinated breathing, as can massage of the lung zones, and gentle dispersed pressure over the heart zone will suppress palpitations. If a mother has had some severe emotional upheaval in the recent past, such as a bereavement or a relationship breakdown, or even an extremely stressful house move, the heart zones may be very red and "angry looking" and may also be tender on palpation. In orthodox terms this may be attributed solely to pressure of the shoes; a reflexology practitioner who is not attuned to the situation may assume that it indicates changed physiology or an actual or impending cardiac condition. However, it is extremely rare that a woman of reproductive years who attends for RZT will have cardiac pathology, and consideration should be given to a history of major emotional trauma, although care should be taken not to overstep professional boundaries. If it is thought that there is a deep-seated emotional problem the mother should, of course, be referred for appropriate counselling.

Manipulative movements to stretch and ease the spine zone can be combined with sedation of zones for the thoracic spine, cardiac sphincter and oesophagus, according to the precise symptoms of the individual mother. The spine zones should also be worked from the cervical vertebrae to the coccyx, usually two or three times, with sedation of any specific areas denoting problems such as upper or lower backache, and the advanced technique can also be employed (see Appendix 2).

It may be appropriate to teach the mother or her partner to sedate the "solar plexus" zone on the hands for use in stressful situations, for example, having blood taken in the antenatal clinic, or awaiting results of specific investigations such as amniocentesis (Stephenson et al 2003). In an acute situation, where the mother experiences panic attacks, *brief* sedation of the adrenal gland zones will reduce the adrenaline levels and restore a more homeostatic balance. This technique should not, however, be used for the treatment of longer-term conditions nor for general anxiety and stress. The practitioner should be able to locate the kidney zones accurately and then tip the thumbs over the top and into the precise areas for the adrenal glands; this should be held for no more than 3–5 seconds, as prolonged pressure may cause further palpitations and trigger nausea.

During pregnancy, many women desire regular treatments and these can be given every 2–3 weeks, then weekly from about 36 weeks' gestation. It is not usually necessary to employ specific sedating or stimulating techniques unless the mother is experiencing symptoms; therefore, a gentle all-over treatment is usually all that is required. There is evidence, within general medicine, to suggest that teaching family members to use touch therapies such as reflexology can ease distress and aid empathy and communication (Collinge et al 2007, Stephenson et al 2007), although no studies have been undertaken on teaching partners to work on pregnant women. However, this may provide an opportunity for the couple to spend time together and for the partner to feel integral to the care in pregnancy.

Although discussed here in relation to pregnancy, the principles of treatment for general relaxation, stress, anxiety, panic and sleep disorders are relevant also in the puerperium (see Chapter 6).

NAUSEA AND VOMITING; HYPERSALIVATION

Structural physiology and aetiology

Nausea and/or vomiting affects up to 85% of pregnant women (Jewell & Young 2003), may persist for much longer than the first trimester and can occur at any time of the day or night, the popular notion of "*morning* sickness" arising from the nausea triggered by hypoglycaemia on waking. Tiredness, hunger, anxiety and multiple pregnancy exacerbate the symptoms, as does a tendency to travel sickness. Symptoms may be accompanied by heartburn, food cravings or aversions, excessive salivation, constipation, diarrhoea or headaches.

Nausea is thought to be due primarily to the hormones, human chorionic gondatotrophin (hCG), oestrogen and progesterone. It can be useful to reassure the mother, since her symptoms are so distressing, that it indicates that she has sufficiently high levels of hormones to sustain the pregnancy. Symptoms may also be due to a deficiency of thyroid stimulating hormone which occurs in response to hCG (Panesar 2001), possibly with accompanying immunological implications (Minagawa 1999). Vomiting is initiated from the vomiting centre in the medulla of the brain, which controls smooth muscle in the stomach wall and skeletal muscle in the abdomen and respiratory centre. This is also responsible for motion sickness and may be exacerbated by changes in the sense of equilibrium (balance) resulting from motion effects on the vestibular apparatus in the ear. If there is any suspicion that infection may be causing the vomiting, for example pyelonephritis or gastroenteritis, RZT should not be performed, especially if the mother is pyrexial. Other pathological causes usually involve excessive vomiting, which should be differentiated from hyperemesis gravidarum, and referred for medical treatment as appropriate. (For an in-depth exploration of complementary therapies for nausea and vomiting see Tiran 2004b.)

From a musculoskeletal perspective, research by this author suggests a very strong correlation between the increased severity of gestational nausea and vomiting and a history of back, neck or jaw problems. Examples include whiplash injury, coccygeal or pelvic trauma from a fall, or jaw misalignment from a fracture or difficult dental surgery, such as extraction of impacted wisdom teeth, and it is, therefore, useful to check the mother's musculoskeletal history (see Chapter 2). Certainly, symptoms will be compounded by the impact of the expanding uterus on the upper gastrointestinal tract and compromised biomechanical movement in the diaphragm, thorax and upper abdomen, whilst tension in the cervical spine may aggravate the vagus nerve, further exacerbating nausea. It is also interesting to note that mothers who experience severe nausea and vomiting in the first and second trimester, attributed to musculoskeletal aetiology, often return for treatment in the third trimester with a breech presentation. This may be due to the altered angle of inclination of the pelvic brim, which prevents the fetal head from entering and remaining in the pelvic cavity, the fetus therefore settling in a more comfortable presentation.

In addition to the nausea and/or vomiting, some women also have associated hypersalivation (ptyalism), which can be severe, requiring them to spit constantly. Hypersalivation is a common feature of pregnancy in women of Afro-Caribbean descent, to the extent that it is considered normal, if distressing, although no physiological explanation can be given for the phenomenon. Occasionally, in Afro-Caribbean and women of other ethnic origin, this may also be related to a previous neck injury, or to problems lower in the spine, such as coccygeal trauma from a fall. Most commonly those with hypersalivation will have had forceful dental surgery or perhaps a previous fracture of the jaw and the practitioner may become aware of this from both the history and the visual and manual examinations of the feet. Conversely, injury or surgery on or near one or both big toes may have left a residual misalignment or misshapen toe, which reflects back to the relevant body area, leading to apparently idiopathic, but actually iatrogenic, problems in the head or neck.

Relevant reflexology treatment

Some expectant mothers with "morning sickness" will not wish to be treated with RZT, although tactile therapies have been shown to be popular as a means of providing respite from unremitting symptoms (Agren & Berg 2006). Women suffering nausea and vomiting are the most likely to experience rapid and profound effects during and after RZT, and prolonged, rapid or excessively forceful treatment may actually trigger nausea. A healing crisis usually occurs within the first 24 hours following therapy, also possibly causing her to feel temporarily worse; she should be informed of this and given the opportunity to decline treatment if she feels that she would be unable to cope with the effects. Using the Likert scale to encourage the mother to assess the severity of her symptoms (see Chapter 2) may help her to recognise the extent to which the RZT treatment has helped to alleviate the nausea, vomiting or other accompanying symptoms.

Once the mother has agreed to receive treatment, it is useful first to assess alignment of the pelvis by measuring the level of the two iliac crests (hip bones), as described in Chapter 2, to identify any possible musculoskeletal indicators. Visual examination of the feet may identify possible contributory factors, giving a guide to relevant treatment. Musculoskeletal misalignment may be indicated by the position of the feet on the couch or the angle of the feet or toes in relation to each other. Observation of the thyroid gland reflex zone may reveal a grey-blue and slightly puffy area, suggesting a thyroid implication to the aetiology (usually a deficiency of thyroxine). More severe problems such as undiagnosed hiatus hernia may be revealed through manual examination, the diaphragm line being felt as an intermittent zone, with the mother experiencing tenderness on being touched. If there is any doubt about the cause or effects of the mother's condition she should not be treated on this occasion; similarly if the practitioner feels unsure or lacks confidence to justify her treatment, further advice should be sought before performing RZT.

A light general relaxation treatment can be given if the mother can tolerate it, with the actual hands-on component (as opposed to the visual examination) lasting *no longer than 20 minutes* to avoid adverse reactions. A systematic all-over treatment should be undertaken; no reflex zones should be avoided but those which are significant to the individual mother's physiology should not be stimulated unless there is an indication to do so. "Solar plexus" pressure should be *extremely light*, no more than merely touching the skin, without any indentation visible; this can be repeated periodically throughout the treatment. However, overworking the relaxation point can induce severe nausea and will necessitate cessation of the treatment. Care should be taken when working on the big toe, the reflex zones for the head and neck, as over-zealous massage can inadvertently stimulate the zone for the vagus nerve, exacerbating nausea. Other relaxation techniques, including "diaphragm sweeping" generalised effleurage of the feet and intermittent holding, should form a major component of treatment by reflexologists who feel cautious about determining and treating the precise cause of the sickness (see Appendix 1).

> It is essential, when treating women with first trimester "morning sickness", that the practitioner understands the individual's physiopathology; extremely cautious treatment, particularly to the "solar plexus" point, is vital to avoid exacerbating the mother's symptoms.

Sedation of specific reflex zones can be useful in some, but not all, women. This may be achieved either through pressure applied to the precise zone, e.g. the stomach, cardiac sphincter and intestines if these are tender, or with a more diversified coverage of these zones by placing the palms of the hands over the generalised area, which is said to restore equilibrium to the autonomic nervous system (Lett 2000:218). Gentle sedation of the thoracic spine may be effective in temporarily calming the neurological triggers to nausea.

Women with longstanding back problems may benefit from manipulation of the bony areas of the feet, which correspond to the spine, shoulders, ribs and pelvis, in an attempt to release tension. It is probable that, in those with a history of whiplash injury or other neck problem, tenderness will be felt by the mother in her big toes, and tension, rigidity or immobility will be felt by the practitioner, depending on the severity of the condition. The advanced technique (see Appendix 2) can be used with care to release some of this tension, but the practitioner must observe the mother's reactions and be prepared to stop if undue reactions occur. This author uses this a very specific technique, developed, adapted and researched over a 15-year period, in which nausea and vomiting may sometimes be treated in a single 10-minute treatment in approximately 65% of women. In the event that a single treatment does not resolve the problem, additional sessions are offered, but if the problem has not improved after the third treatment, this approach is not appropriate and alternative means of helping the mother are used (such as homeopathy, hypnotherapy or referral for osteopathy or acupuncture). Treatments should be given approximately every 5–7 days; it is not appropriate to give them more frequently since the mother's body requires time to respond to and adapt to the effects of the treatment (see Fig. 4.1).

Sedation of the thyroid zone should *never* be performed in pregnancy, even when it appears or feels abnormal, since this could interfere with the functioning of the organ. Similarly, stimulation is not always appropriate as it is impossible to determine the "dose" given, with a consequent risk of over-stimulation. The practitioner should investigate whether the mother has had blood taken for thyroid function, whether she has already been prescribed thyroid medication; she must also investigate whether any visual

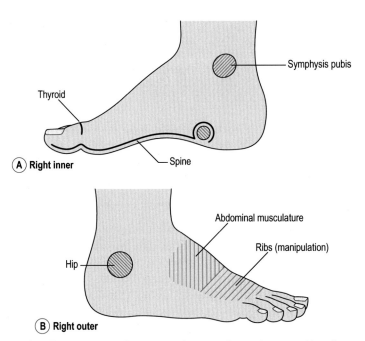

Fig 4.1   Treatment zones for nausea and vomiting, hypersalivation and heartburn; (A) right inner, (B) right outer, (C) sole (right), (D) dorsum (left)

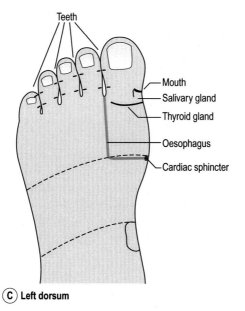

Teeth

Mouth
Salivary gland
Thyroid gland

Oesophagus
Cardiac sphincter

C **Left dorsum**

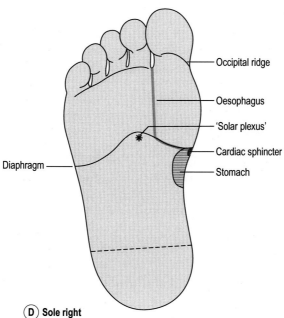

Occipital ridge

Oesophagus

'Solar plexus'

Cardiac sphincter

Stomach

Diaphragm

D **Sole right**

Fig. 4.1 cont'd

irregularities in the thyroid foot zone could be coincidental. *No* specific treatment should be performed on this zone if the mother is taking thyroid medication.

In the event of hyperemesis gravidarum gentle relaxation treatment is permissible with caution, once major pathological causes have been eliminated, with light sedation of the reflex zones for the endocrine system and gastrointestinal tract.

CASE STUDY 4.1 NAUSEA AND VOMITING

Maria, a mature student of architecture at a local university, attended the complementary therapy midwife's clinic at 17 weeks' gestation with a history of constant nausea and frequent vomiting since 6 weeks of pregnancy. On entering the clinic her face was observed to be grey and pale, her posture was hunched as if she was very cold and she appeared introspective, miserable and depressed with a rather hopeless attitude to her symptoms.

During the history taking, she reported that she had had a car accident about 2 years before and suffered a whiplash injury, which still occasionally gave her pain, especially when she spent long hours at the computer or doing close work such as drawing. On examination of her feet, the big toes (neck zones) were darkly shaded all round and there were marked creases on their plantar surfaces in the areas corresponding to the occiput. She felt considerable pain when these toes were touched and initially could hardly bear the midwife to work on them.

After a few minutes of calming and relaxing movements on the feet, the practitioner felt that Maria would be able to tolerate more manipulative work. The big toes were extremely stiff and rigid, with palpable ridges on the occipital zones. The midwife used the advanced technique (Appendix 2), with traction and careful outwards rotation and felt impaired movement beneath her working fingers which gradually responded to further manipulation.

The result was astounding. After only 2 minutes the first big toe suddenly eased with an audible "crack" and a palpable release of tension; the plantar ridge seemed to reduce in prominence and the overall rigidity disappeared. The mother immediately sat up straight, her face became pink and she started smiling and chatting. Further work on the second big toe was minimal and Maria was able, after a few minutes' rest, almost to spring off the couch and to walk out of the clinic looking much more lively and happy. She did not need another appointment and follow-up with her own midwife revealed that her symptoms had totally resolved, instantaneously and apparently permanently, enabling her to progress through a normal pregnancy with no further problems.

If the mother is also experiencing hypersalivation, sedation of the relevant reflex zones will be necessary. On the dorsal surface of the two big toes the area which relates to the reflex zone for the jaw is near the reflex zone for the mouth and, with careful palpation, will be found to be tender; sometimes there will be a sensation of misshapen bone formation or misaligned bone healing, and this will tend to feel bruised when pressed. The salivary gland reflex zones are fractionally distal and inferior to those for the mouth and run down to the base of the dorsal surface of the big toe. Locating the epicentre of the relevant area and using a sedating technique usually provides some relief, albeit temporary, and the mother can be shown the corresponding area on the thumbs, for self-treatment at home. The advanced manipulative technique can be employed if the practitioner feels that there is tension in the big toes, plus palpation of the wisdom teeth zones on the medial aspect of the fifth toes may indicate a need for treatment here. Traction and rotation should be applied gently and carefully, observing the mother for any adverse reactions, including pain, nausea or dizziness. Usually, application of slight traction followed by a sharp pulling of the toes will ease any rigidity, although in the case of previous impacted wisdom teeth or difficult extractions there may be a ridge of bone felt in the reflex zone on the medial aspect of the little toe as a result of posterior jaw misalignment (see Fig. 4.1).

It is also important to treat other concomitant symptoms, such as heartburn, constipation or headaches, which should not be viewed in isolation, but may be directly related to the presenting problem. This will include sedating and/or stimulating techniques as appropriate (see relevant sections). Alleviation of some of these accompanying symptoms may help the mother to cope better with the nausea, vomiting and hypersalivation, with a consequent reduction in her perception of the overall severity of her condition, as assessed on the Likert scale.

CASE STUDY 4.2   HYPERSALIVATION

Adebayo was a Nigerian anaesthetist who reported to the complementary therapy midwife's clinic with excessive salivation at 12 weeks' gestation in her first pregnancy. Although she accepted that this was a common and normal pregnancy symptom, especially amongst her own race, she was finding it very difficult to cope and needed to carry a pot with her into which she could spit the copious amounts of saliva which she was producing. She had taken time off from work as it was even more difficult to cope when masked up in the operating theatre.

There was no relevant pathological history, nor any noticeable disorder of the foot reflex zones on visual examination. However, on palpation, the midwife found that the dorsal surface of one big toe was swollen, with a significant energy pulsating from it and "grittiness" under the skin in the area corresponding to the mouth and salivary glands. She applied sedating techniques at first and then used the advanced technique, applying traction and rotation to the toe until it released. She also worked on the cervical vertebrae zones where there was some rigidity. After the first treatment Adebayo felt a little better and had stopped needing to carry the pot with her. After a further two treatments the hypersalivation had subsided to a manageable level and she was able to return to work.

Early in her second pregnancy Adebayo again started experiencing symptoms and attended the clinic for reflexology. Two treatments were all that were required, at weeks 8 and 9, and this time she did not have to take time off from work. She was so impressed with the treatment that she proceeded to recommend it, over the next few years, to other Nigerian medical colleagues suffering gestational hypersalivation who then attended the clinic with similar results!

HEADACHES AND MIGRAINE; NECK PAIN

Structural physiology and aetiology

Headaches are a common phenomenon in the first trimester due to the increased circulating blood volume and the dilatory effects of progesterone on the cerebral blood vessels. In the absence of any known pathology, headaches may be related to tiredness, stress or anxiety about a variety of physical, emotional or social/occupational issues; rarely does the symptom arise in isolation. Headaches may also be triggered by dehydration, "morning sickness" and constipation; these are often felt in the base of the occipital region. In the third trimester they may herald the onset of fulminating pre-eclampsia, particularly frontal headaches, as a result of oedema around the brain and the optic nerve (although an eye test may reveal ophthalmic problems in the case of pain directly over the eyes). Third trimester headaches should never be ignored; therapists who are not midwives must refer the mother back to her conventional maternity care team.

Structurally, any injury, disease or genetic or acquired problem which affects the back and/or neck will also, at some time, impact higher up the spine, and this is especially likely during pregnancy when the neighbouring ligaments and joints are relaxed through the action of relaxin. Women who spend long hours hunched over a computer may already have suffered headaches prior to conception and these may become more frequent or severe during pregnancy. Previous neck or head injury may have caused the woman to make subconscious compensatory adjustments in her posture and movement, but the relaxation of joints and ligaments in pregnancy often causes pain to recur, albeit temporarily. Commonly, these women will also report, when questioned, suffering pain elsewhere, including the upper back, notably between the scapulae, across the shoulder girdle, sometimes also involving the arms and hands, or frontally above the xiphisternum. Conversely, headaches may occur only as pregnancy progresses and may be linked to increased weight, especially breast enlargement, which puts additional stress on the cervical vertebrae.

The aetiology of chronic headaches and migraine is complex and may occasionally relate to serious pathology, such as hypertension or renal disease, although women with pre-existing conditions will normally be aware of these and may already be receiving medical treatment. Women who have suffered migraines before conception may experience a worsening of their symptoms during pregnancy, particularly if they are hormonal in origin or if they have been forced to stop or change their medication, although this is not universal. Migraine which persists through pregnancy may also be accompanied by nausea and vomiting or by disruption to the bowels, triggered through neurological and vascular links.

Relevant reflexology treatment

Simple "first aid" treatment to reduce the symptoms can be achieved through sedation of the relevant areas of the reflex zones for the head and neck. Palpation of the entire surface of the toes on both feet will elicit the location of any tender spots which indicate the areas to be treated. Sedation, by sustained pressure applied to the limit of the mother's tolerance level, may reduce or eliminate the tenderness on the feet, which in turn will ease the headache. Sedation may be required for several minutes in severe cases and most clients report that, although the pain does not always vanish completely, the overall pain is dissipated and diluted to a manageable level, relief which may last for an hour or two. If there is any neck involvement, the advanced manipulative technique (Appendix 2) can be administered to release tensions in the spinal vertebrae, diaphragm and associated muscles. Headache caused by dehydration may respond to sedation of the reflex zone for the occiput and neighbouring structures, and the mother should also, obviously, be advised to increase her fluid intake.

Stimulating techniques are not appropriate for this symptom as they would result in an exacerbation of the problem. It is also necessary to be aware of any underlying pathology and to rationalise the specific techniques used: sedation should not, for example, be applied to the precise point for the pituitary gland zone (see Chapter 2). Caution should also be taken when working on the reflex zones for the neck, as over-stimulation could trigger nausea or exacerbate symtoms already present.

Longer-term resolution may be achieved through general relaxation RZT sessions, which incorporate relevant manipulative techniques (see Appendix 2). These relaxation treatments will not necessarily eliminate the cause if there is a related medical condition, such as hypertension, although mild to moderate hypertension may be alleviated with regular treatments, especially if stress-induced (McVicar et al 2007). Unfortunately, however, time and financial constraints may influence the provision and effectiveness of RZT for chronic headaches and migraines which require regular, frequent and, possibly, long-term treatments.

HEARTBURN AND INDIGESTION

Structural physiology and aetiology

Heartburn, indigestion and acid reflux all commonly occur in pregnancy, usually in the latter stage, although they may also accompany first trimester nausea and vomiting. Symptoms are largely due to the effects of progesterone, which relaxes the cardiac sphincter of the stomach, causing acid reflux. It is worse in women with multiple pregnancy and when the fetal presentation is breech, due to upwards pressure on the diaphrgam. Some mothers may experience a burning sensation at varying levels in the oesophagus, which will usually correspond to tender areas on the oesophagus reflex zones of the feet, relative to the level of heartburn. Mechanical distress also occurs at the junction of the oesophagus, cardiac sphincter and stomach due to changes within the abdominal/uterine cavities, the spinal kyphosis/lordosis and the inter-relationship between the shoulder and pelvic girdles. Heartburn is also often exacerbated by the weight of the breasts, particularly if the mother wears an ill-fitting brassiere, or if her general posture is poor with an accentuated thoracic kyphosis.

Relevant reflexology treatment

During the exploratory phase of the treatment session the mother may report tenderness in the zones for the oesophagus, with a general bruised sensation along the entire zone and a sharp, burning pain at the precise location of the symptom. Asking her to indicate on her chest exactly where she feels the heartburn most profoundly will also enable the practitioner to "home in" on the specific location on the mother's feet. The strongest indicators will be found on the dorsal surface of the feet, in keeping with the possible existence of an "indirect" zone for the oesophagus (see Chapter 3), whereas one might expect it to be on the plantar surface. Very precise sedation of this point can be performed, as well as on the cardiac sphincter zone. Care should be taken not to sedate the stomach zone, as opposed to the minute area corresponding to the cardiac sphincter, as this may interfere with normal physiology in the stomach and it is not the intention to suppress acid production, merely to reduce reflux. The mother can also be shown the relevant zones for the oesophagus on the hands and directed to simple "first aid" sedation of the points if the symptoms become troublesome at night (see Fig. 4.1).

Structural RZT techniques include the manipulation of the medial aspect of the foot corresponding to the thoracic cavity, diaphragm sweeping to calm the diaphragmatic spasm and gentle work over the zones for the abdominal musculature on the lower dorsum of each foot. Additionally, the advanced technique (Appendix 2) may help to release tension and rigidity in the cervical vertebrae, which can impact lower down the spine, and working the reflex zones of the shoulders may relieve tension due to heavy breasts.

CONSTIPATION

Structural physiology and aetiology

Constipation is common in pregnancy as progesterone relaxes the intestines, slowing peristalsis. It is worsened by poor diet, inadequate fluid intake, lack of exercise and some iron tablets, and may accompany gestational nausea and vomiting, or irritable bowel syndrome, in combination with diarrhoea. The diagnosis is somewhat subjective, being based on a reduction in frequency of defaecation compared to normal, altered consistency of the stool, difficulty in passing the stool, palpable stools in the rectum and, in severe cases, faecal soiling with overflow. Physically these symptoms may be due to poor diet and/or fluid intake, reduced gut motility or an altered sensation of the need to defaecate (often associated with haemorrhoids in pregnancy or perineal and anal trauma immediately postnatally), but may be exacerbated by discomfort, embarrassment or fear of pain.

Pelvic congestion from downwards pressure of the uterus in late pregnancy can also add to the general discomfort. Weakness of abdominal and pelvic floor musculature will exacerbate the problem, creating neural irritation and disordered enteric coordination. Since peristaltic movement is affected by vagus nerve activity, any factor affecting vagal function will also predispose a woman to more severe constipation than normal. This may, for example, be related to problems in the upper cervical spine or the occipital ridge. Disordered sacrococcygeal mechanics will affect, or may be caused by, tension on the uterus and uterosacral ligaments and will indirectly affect circulation in the rectum. Some women experience accompanying backache, possibly related to additional deviations within the spine, or more local discomfort as a result of straining at stool, and pain in the coccygeal area is common. Osteopaths believe that there is an embryological link between the coccyx and the ethmoid bone in the anterior skull at the roof of the nose (Stone 2007:306) and that, therefore, any misalignment of one will affect the other.

Relevant reflexology treatment

Basic RZT aims to stimulate peristalsis, so the simplest treatment involves *clockwise* massage of the arches of the feet, the areas relating to the intestines. More precise treatment can be performed on the zones for the entire gastrointestinal tract, from the reflex zones for the mouth to the oesophagus and stomach, large and small intestines and on to the rectum and anal sphincter zones. Sedation of the pelvic floor reflex zones may be helpful, especially in the early puerperium if the mother has concomitant haemorrhoids. A useful "tip" is to advise mothers with constipation to try rolling a bottle under the arch of each foot whilst sitting in a chair in the evenings, as this also applies stimulation to the intestinal reflex zones. In an attempt to stimulate the general metabolism, the zone for the liver can also be specifically stimulated, although, in practice, this occurs indirectly through working on the intestinal zones on the right plantar surface. Stimulating techniques can also be used on the abdominal musculature on the dorsum of the feet.

If the mother reports accompanying backache a careful exploration of the zones for the spine can be made and any relevant areas can be sedated. Special attention should be given to the cervical vertebral zone; if tension is felt in the big toes, the advanced neck release technique (Appendix 2) should be used. Gentle manipulative movements may be effective in releasing musculoskeletal tension which may be contributing to misalignment and consequent tension on the gut. Also, any restriction in the coccyx may adversely affect the mechanism of defaecation in the rectum and anus, causing inhibitory faecal retention. The link between the coccyx and the ethmoid bone suggests that manipulative movements should include the face, and it is interesting to note that some women with constipation also complain of sinus congestion. However, if the mother has irritable bowel syndrome (IBS) with intermittent constipation, care should be taken not to over-stimulate the spinal reflex zones which may trigger the diarrhoeic phase of the condition. If the IBS is exacerbated by stress, a course of general relaxation sessions may be the treatment of choice (see Fig. 4.2).

HAEMORRHOIDS

Structural physiology and aetiology

Haemorrhoids, like other varicose veins, develop in susceptible pregnant women as a result of the relaxation effect of the progesterone on smooth muscles. Mothers may experience itching and pain, and the haemorrhoids may prolapse or start to bleed slightly, most commonly after a bowel motion. Excessive weight gain, multiple pregnancy and repeated pregnancies will

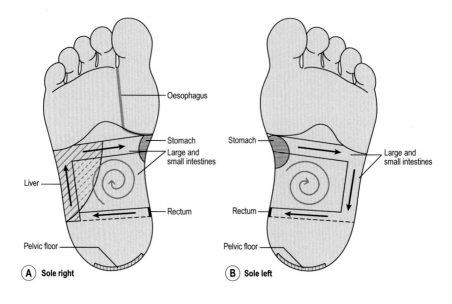

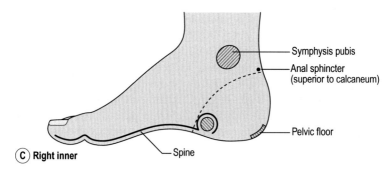

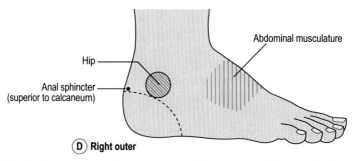

Fig 4.2   Treatment zones for constipation and haemorrhoids; (A) right sole, (B) left sole, (C) right inner, (D) right outer

increase the likelihood of haemorrhoids, as will poor diet, smoking and irregular bowels habits or constipation. Women who have suffered haemorrhoids prior to or between pregnancies are much more prone to problems in the current pregnancy.

Musculoskeletal factors which affect venous drainage, together with deviations in the spine impacting on the diaphragm and thorax, will potentially contribute to, or encourage, the development of haemorrhoids. Venous drainage is via the portal system of the liver, then from the liver to the inferior vena cava and systemic circulation. If the filtering system of the liver becomes congested it will lead to compression and torsion in the veins nearest the organ, impairing bloodflow from the gut to the inferior vena cava. The consequent damming effect causes varicosities anywhere along the gastrointestinal tract, presenting most commonly in pregnancy as problems such as haemorrhoids. (In severe cases, mostly in non-pregnant patients, there may be oesophageal varices.) Further, any misalignment affecting the diaphragm or ribcage may exacerbate the problem, because these exert a "sucking" motion to assist in the mechanics of the portal circulation and general venous drainage, thus aiding the return of fluid from the abdomen and legs to the thorax.

Relevant reflexology treatment

The indirect zones for the anal sphincter (see Chapter 3) will feel tender to touch; this is the part of the foot, just above the heel, where the Achilles tendon is situated. Tenderness may be felt on both the medial and distal sides of this area, or may be unilateral; discomfort will be more pronounced if the haemorrhoids are bleeding or prolapsed. Occasionally this area will feel uncomfortable to touch even before the mother has experienced symptoms of haemorrhoids, notably if she has had them in a previous pregnancy, when the sensation will be a bruised feeling. However, this facilitates the practitioner to offer relevant dietary advice to avoid constipation in an attempt to reduce the severity of the impending haemorrhoids.

Since constipation puts undue pressure on the haemorrhoids at defaecation the anal sphincter zone cannot be treated in isolation, although a simple first-aid sedation of the area will provide immediate, albeit temporary, relief. The entire gastrointestinal tract should be treated, with stimulation to the intestinal zones to regulate peristalsis and prevent or reduce the severity of accompanying constipation. It can also be useful to sedate the pelvic floor reflex zones, taking care not to apply pressure inadvertently to the uterus zone. Manipulative techniques can also be used on the spine reflex zones to aid adjustment and realignment and stimulation of the abdominal musculature zones may aid relaxation of the entire lower trunk. Careful stimulation of the liver zone may also be necessary, although in practice, this is usually covered when working over the reflex zones for the intestines (Fig. 4.2).

CASE STUDY 4.3 CONSTIPATION AND HAEMORRHOIDS

Izzie presented to the complementary therapies (CT) midwifery clinic with a history of constipation throughout the 29 weeks of her second pregnancy, with irregular, infrequent and ineffective bowel movements.

Continued

Her last labour had been prolonged due to a persistent occipito-posterior position. The delivery of the baby, who weighed 4.3 kg, was extremely difficult and resulted in shoulder dystocia and a fractured coccyx; the baby had been born with an Apgar score of 3, but had recovered and was now a healthy 3-year-old. Izzie had tried dietary measures for her constipation and resorted to laxatives occasionally but with no real effect. She had gained a lot of weight so far in this pregnancy and reported dragging abdominal and perineal sensations and tenderness in the coccyx; she also suspected she was developing haemorrhoids.

The CT midwife examined Izzie's feet and was immediately struck by a dark purple, bruise-like lesion on the part of the left foot relating to the coccyx which, when pressed, felt very tender. Izzie also reported a sharp pain in the indirect zone for the anal sphincter, and when the midwife palpated the arches of the feet, they felt very bloated and congested, and had a mottled appearance. On the first reflex zone therapy (RZT) treatment Izzie could only tolerate some gentle relaxation techniques and firm clockwise massage of the reflex zones for the intestines, plus sedation of the zones for the coccyx and anus. The following week, there had been no real progress, but the arches of the feet looked less mottled. The midwife was able to use manipulative techniques and elicited some audible "cracks" in the big toes when working on the zones for the cervical vertebrae, but the coccygeal zone remained tender and "angry looking". Sedation of the anal sphincter zone was repeated and was less tender than previously.

On the third treatment, Izzie reported that her constipation was no better and that she had had several nose bleeds during the week, which, although common in pregnancy, had not affected her before; the midwife sedated the reflex zones for the nose, and repeated the relaxation and manipulative treatment, including the advanced technique on the big toe and sedation of the reflex zone for the coccyx, which was now less painful. By the fourth week, Izzie looked and felt much better; the haemorrhoids were less painful and no longer bleeding, the nose bleeds had not recurred and she had had two good bowel movements during the week. The abdominal dragging sensation had lessened and the coccygeal pain had receded; amazingly, the reflex zone for the coccyx was no longer tender, and had changed to a light bluish colour, which was hardly noticeable. Izzie now felt able to tackle the constipation by herself and she did not need any further treatments.

BACKACHE, SCIATICA AND SYMPHYSIS PUBIS DISCOMFORT

Structural physiology and aetiology

Musculoskeletal discomforts cause considerable distress to women throughout pregnancy, adversely affecting their daily lives and impacting on the family. Chronic spinal or pelvic problems can be completely debilitating and may also contribute to psychological distress, leading to stress and depression (Field et al 2006). The conventional explanation for backache and associated symptoms in pregnancy is the effect of the hormones, relaxin and progesterone, on the joints, ligaments and muscles in and around the spine and pelvis, causing increased lumbar lordosis, and an altered centre of gravity due to weight gain, which is distributed anteriorly. In structural terms, there is considerable force during pregnancy directed through the uterosacral ligaments, whilst the weight of the enlarging uterus is taken by the pelvic floor, which affects sacroiliac, coccygeal, pubic and lumbosacral joint movement. Increasing weight and pressure as pregnancy progresses further stresses the uterosacral ligaments causing back pain in many women. If the changes required in the spinal curves to assist rotation of the pelvic girdle (as described in Chapter 1) do not occur smoothly, there is additional mechanical stress in the lumbar vertebrae which eventually causes irritation of the surrounding soft tissues, particularly in late pregnancy. If there is excessive extension at the lumbosacral junction the weight is transferred to articulating joints nearby, which are not designed for this function, therefore spasm, inflammation and tension accumulate and cause pain and impaired movement. Furthermore, the ligaments between the lumbar region and the ilium may become affected by poor mechanics in the sacral and lumbar areas, causing irritation and pain as a result of uneven (unilateral) tension.

Pre-existing misalignment of the musculoskeletal system will aggravate the discomfort, as will incoordinate ergonomics, such as an accentuated posture when sitting at a computer. Poor abdominal muscle tone, which supports the thoracic and lumbar spine, and, later in pregnancy, relaxation of the pelvic floor also contribute to the problem. Women with a history of slipped discs in the lumbar region are, understandably, at greater risk of severe pain in pregnancy, as are those who have previously had spinal surgery or coccygeal trauma.

Several types of musculoskeletal pain occur during pregnancy, including lumbosacral, symphysis pubis discomfort, unilateral or bilateral sacroiliac joint pain, sciatica or a combination of two or more. Other problems, such as carpal tunnel syndrome, shoulder and upper back pain, knee pain and headaches, are often assoicated with instability of the pelvic girdle.

Pelvic girdle syndrome is defined as pain in all three major joint areas and is considered to have a far worse prognosis than pain resulting from one area only (Nilsson-Wikmar et al 1999). The biomechnical changes in the lower back and limbs resulting from the increasing weight may compound relaxin-induced joint instability. Tension and misalignment in the lower limb(s) affect the hip girdle, and cause undue stress on the sacroiliac joints and/or symphysis pubis. A change in the angle of inclination of the pelvic brim leads to lumbosacral extension and stress in other vertebrae, with subsequent pain; excessive elasticity in the sacroiliac ligaments and/or poor pelvic floor tone will place additional strain on the joints, ligaments and muscles. Symphysis pubis discomfort is an increasingly common problem in pregnancy, possibly related to more sedentary lifestyles than previously; the instability of the entire pelvis may be directed forwards in some women, causing increased laxity of the anterior pelvic joints and ligaments. Poor tone elsewhere, such as the rectus abdominis and psoas muscles aggravate pain, whilst compression or irritation of the sciatic nerve may cause sciatica.

Neural tension and movement may be affected by abnormal movement of the head, neck, thoracic cage and lumbar spine, also contributing to sciatica, and displacement of the uterus as it enlarges, or by other organs as they adapt to the growing uterus may add further pressure to the nerves. Sciatic nerve irritation and posterior pelvic pain may also be caused by piriformis syndrome (Papadopoulos & Khan 2004), in which the piriformis muscle is adversely affected by distortion of the hips and sacrum, affecting the neural plexus in the sacrum and/or the sciatic nerve directly.

Coccygeal pain may ensue from tension in the sacroiliac, ischiosacral and coccygeal ligaments triggered by the altered pelvic angle, joint mobility and abnormal rotation of the femoral head in the acetabulum. Pelvic floor and levator ani tension and the impact of the uterine weight on the uterosacral ligaments influence coccygeal and sacral mechanics and cause local pain and irritation. Weakness, tension or scarring of the pelvic floor muscles may distort the coccygeal alignment, which in turn can affect rectal circulation or exacerbate haemorrhoids, another source of pain in the coccyx.

Relevant reflexology treatment

The mother may need to be assisted onto the couch: a stool or small step is a useful aid. The practitioner should ensure that the mother does not overly abduct her legs as she climbs onto the couch, which may need to be lowered until she is in position. Attention should be given to ensuring that she is completely comfortable on the couch before treatment commences.

Visual examination may reveal focus points along the reflex zone for the spine; swelling around one or both of the hip reflex zones, a brownish discolouration under the reflex zone for the symphysis pubis and/or blueness or puffiness on the indirect zones for the knees. After intial relaxation movements, specific RZT work can be performed, focusing on the spine, ribs, pelvis and abdominal muscle reflex zones, but also incorporating any reflex zones which appear to be disordered. The spine should always be worked from the zone for the first cervical vertebra downwards to determine the areas which require treatment. It is worth noting that the area of the spine at which the mother reports pain may not necessarily correspond to the location of significant findings on the spine reflex zone, e.g. the mother may be experiencing lumbosacral pain, yet the causative reflex zone is found to be in the thoracic region. In these cases, both areas should be worked, with a sedating technique at first. Diaphragm "sweeping" is also useful, as is manipulation and massage of the zones for the scapulae, which often display signs of severe muscular tension as a reaction to the altered positioning.

Later, the manipulative movements can be incorporated into the treatment. As the entire musculoskeletal system is interconnected, treatment must be given to all zones corresponding to the bones, joints, ligaments and muscles, as well as those for lymphatic drainage. The advanced technique may help to relieve neck tension, the twisting and "push-pull" movement over the ribcage zones and ankle circling to aid pelvic movement. When working on the big toes, it may also help to apply gentle sustained pressure to the zones for the occiput, especially if the mother complains of headaches. These reflex zones may be felt as ridges on the plantar surface of the big toes, sometimes more prominent on one foot than the other. The zones may initially be immensely painful to touch, but pain usually reduces with gentle massage of the occipital zones and this appears to improve pain lower down the spine. Work on the dorsum, over the area corresponding to the abdominal musculature may need to be stimulating as opposed to sedating, in order to encourage improvement in muscle tone.

If the mother complains of sciatica the outer ankle bone, the zone for the hip, is likely to be swollen on the affected side, potentially making treatment both more uncomfortable for the mother and more difficult for the practitioner. The sacroiliac joint reflex zones and the sciatic nerve zones can be sedated; it is essential to define accurately the location of the sacroiliac joint reflex zone to avoid inadvertently stimulating the Bladder 60 acupressure point (see Chapters 3 and 5). The easiest way to sedate the sciatic nerve zone is to press the length of one finger up the entire zone; this is also usually more comfortable for the mother. Gentle manipulation, including ankle rotations, can be used in an attempt to release tension and restricted musculature, and it will normally be appropriate to sedate the other pelvic joint zones, notably the sacroiliac joints. As with lumbosacral back pain, stimulation of the abdominal musculature may tone up the supporting muscles and provide overall relief.

In the event of symphysis pubis pain the lower 180° of the inner ankle bone may be shaded a brownish, greyish colour and will be tender to the touch. Treatment is best done by sweeping with a finger or thumb around this 180° until the most tender spot is located; sedation can then be applied to the epicentre of this painful spot. In practice, it is often advisable to treat the entire musculoskeletal system, as outlined above, since each part is so closely linked and additional symptoms often develop as the original symptom worsens or is prolonged. Many women will report that they have associated symptoms such as headaches, constipation, stress incontinence or divarification of the rectus sheath and these should also be treated (see relevant sections) (Fig. 4.3).

OEDEMA AND CARPAL TUNNEL SYNDROME

Structural physiology and aetiology

Tingling in the arms and fingers, often accompanied by pain and reduced coordination, is common in pregnancy and is thought to be due to compression by oedema of the nerves in the carpal tunnel running through the wrist. Structurally, the clavicle, scapula, thoracic cavity, anterior chest wall and the junction of the cervical vertebrae with the shoulder girdle may be misaligned. This may be due to previous trauma to the neck, upper back, shoulders or arms, or even to lower back injury resulting in fusion of the lumbosacral vertebrae and consequent hypermobility in the thoracic or cervical vertebrae. Increasing breast size is a significant factor in carpal tunnel syndrome and the mother should be advised to be fitted properly for a well-supporting brassiere. A family or personal history of the problem increases the likelihood of

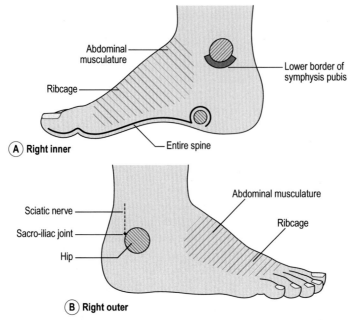

Fig 4.3   Treatment zones for backache, sciatica and symphysis pubis discomfort; (A) right inner, (B) right outer

the condition developing, and although most women find that it resolves spontaneously within a few weeks of delivery, occasionally surgery is required at a later stage.

Relevant reflexology treatment

The foot zones for the hand, forearm, elbow, upper arm, shoulder and neck should all be treated. Sedation may be necessary on the hand zone before any other treatment, and the mother can be shown the hand reflexology point so that she can perform "first aid" treatment at home. Sweeping movements on the zones from the hand to the shoulder will aid drainage of excess fluid back into the circulation, in the same way as generalised massage would be performed up the arm from hand to shoulder. The axillary lymph zones should be drained, using a pinching, sweeping motion, as can those for the head and neck. Manipulation of the scapulae, head and neck zones, as well as the twisting movements of the ribcage zones should be performed, and it is wise to treat the whole of the spine zones, from cervical to coccygeal vertebrae.

Oedema of the ankles and legs is sometimes difficult to treat with RZT, as the use of specific techniques may be too painful for the mother to tolerate. However, a single-blind study by Mollart (2003) compared rest, relaxation reflexology and a specific lymphatic drainage form of reflexology and, although there was no discernible difference in leg circumference between the groups, those who received the lymphatic drainage treatment reported feeling more comfortable. General bimanual stroking (effleurage massage) may assist in directing the fluid back towards the heart. It is useful also to employ drainage techniques to all the lymphatic zones, and to stimulate the renal tract zones. The aim of this is not to increase diuresis but to facilitate a return to homeostasis in the renal tract to encourage fluid in the tissues to return to the kidneys and to be excreted. However, care should be taken if the mother has a history of pre-eclampsia or essential hypertension; if there is any suggestion that the oedema heralds the onset of fulminating pre-eclampsia, RZT should be withheld. The mother may also find it helpful to perform the "wrist wringing" movement as this will assist in drainage of the pelvic lymphatics (see Fig. 4.4).

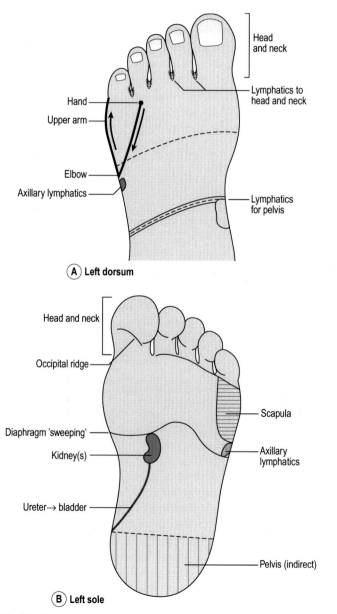

Fig 4.4   Treatment zones for carpal tunnel and oedema; (A) left dorsum, (B) left sole

SINUS CONGESTION

Structural physiology and aetiology

Sinus congestion is a common complaint in pregnancy, although it is often ignored by conventional doctors or considered irrelevant to pregnancy physiology. However, increased vascularity and the vasodilatory effect of progesterone stimulate receptors in the nose and related sinuses of the skull, causing excess mucus to be produced. Chinese medical practitioners deem sinus congestion, chronic coughs and breathlessness to be due to an imbalance in Kidney *chi* (the internal life force passing through the Kidney meridian). Structurally, sinus function can be affected by mechanical tension in the head and neck, which may worsen in pregnancy under the influence of progesterone and relaxin on the upper spine. There is an intimate relationship between the facial structures, respiratory function, mechanics in the throat and posture and position of joints, muscles and ligaments. Mechanical tensions in the shoulders and upper ribs can interfere with the nerve supply to the head and neck as it passes from the upper dorsal segments of the spinal cord and through the thoracic and cervical regions.

Relevant reflexology treatment

"First aid" treatment may consist of stimulating massage of the reflex zones for the facial sinuses and nose: the mother should be forewarned that she may experience a dripping and "runny" nose. Slight stimulation of the "solar plexus" relaxation point, which corresponds to the acupuncture point Kidney 1, may also help the problem as it will provide stimulation to the beginning of the Kidney meridian, thus helping to rebalance Kidney *chi*. Manipulative techniques include applying traction to the reflex zones for the neck, pulling of each toe by grasping it firmly at the base, and bimanual torsion of the shoulder and rib reflex zones. Drainage of the zones for the head and neck lymphatics may also be helpful.

BREECH PRESENTATION

Structural physiology and aetiology

When the fetal breech is the presenting part this can cause problems for delivery. Although fetal presentation and position change frequently during pregnancy, it is expected that most will settle into a cephalic presentation from about 34 weeks' gestation. Thus, although difficulties are not normally encountered until labour, any management or attempt to encourage the fetus to alter position needs to be undertaken in late pregnancy.

There are many reasons why a fetus may adopt a breech presentation: the maternal pelvis may be an abnormal shape, size or in an abnormal position; there may be an obstruction within the uterine cavity, for example placenta praevia, fibroids or another fetus; the fetus/fetal head may be too large. Alternatively, or additionally, there may be loss of muscle tone in either the mother or fetus, as a result of an impaired immune system. This prevents maintenance of a cephalic presentation, since increases in stress hormones such as cortisol, which occur in immunological compromise, impact on prostaglandin production, thereby adversely affecting muscle tone of the maternal uterus and of the fetus (Choi et al 2004).

Conventional management usually consists of offering the mother an external cephalic version (ECV), which is an attempt to turn the fetus by use of external abdominal massage, or a Caesarean section. Vaginal breech birth is rarely offered as obstetricians consider it too risky for mother or baby, although this is debatable.

In structural terms, a misaligned pelvis and spine can alter the angle of inclination of the pelvic brim, making it difficult for the fetal head to enter the pelvis. This may be due to any musculoskeletal trauma, injury or congenital deviation from the normal shape or position of the pelvis or spinal column. Chiropractors acknowledge this misalignment and use a specific manipulation, the Webster technique (Pistolese 2002).

Relevant reflexology treatment

Contrary to the claims of numerous reflexologists (personal communications), reflexology *does not* directly convert a breech presentation to cephalic, as there is no specific "zone" for the fetal position. It would be inappropriate to massage the reflex zone for the uterus in an attempt to encourage the fetus to turn, as this could, theoretically, trigger haemorrhage, placental separation and entanglement of the fetus in the cord. On the other hand, RZT may indirectly help to turn the breech to cephalic, simply by relaxing the mother, aiding homeostasis, stimulating immunological function and improving muscle tone in both the maternal uterus and the fetus. Manipulation of reflex zones for the entire muscusloskeletal system may assist in realigning any deviations which may be contributing to an altered angle of inclination of the pelvic brim, facilitating a change of presentation. This should specifically focus on manipulation and release of tension in the neck and head, bimanual torsion of the rib cage zones and the thoracic spine, toning of the lumbar and sacral spine zones, and treating any discomforts in the system, such as sacroiliac joint, hip or symphysis pubis pain.

Some complementary therapists perform stimulation of a point on the little toes which is often successful in turning the fetus to cephalic. However, this is *not* a reflexology point, but an acupressure point on the feet, the Bladder 67 point, usually stimulated with moxibustion (a heat source used in Chinese medicine). There is considerable literature and research on this increasingly popular technique which is purported to be at least 66% successful (see Tiran 2004a, 2009, van den Berg et al 2008), and is normally performed from 34 weeks' gestation. It is permissible for midwives and reflexologists who fully understand the individual mother's case history to incorporate Bladder 67 acupressure stimulation in an RZT treatment. The fetal presentation must be confirmed by abdominal palpation or by ultrasound scan immediately prior to commencing the course of treatment, the fetal heart should be auscultated before and after the session, and the mother's notes must specify the precise nature of the treatment and any relevant after care (see Chapter 5 and Fig. 5.2 for precise location of the Bladder 67 acupoint).

On no account should stimulation of the Bladder 67 acupoint be performed in women with a history of a previous Caesarean section or other uterine surgery, as treatment may over-stress the scar tissue. Similarly, women with major medical problems such as hypertension, epilepsy, cardiac disease or unstable diabetes should not be treated, nor should those with obstetric complications including multiple pregnancy, placenta praevia, antepartum haemorrhage, or any mother who is due to have a planned Caesarean section for a specific medical reason. Any mother who has been informed by her obstetrician or midwife that an ECV is not appropriate for her personal medical condition should not be treated with Bladder 67 stimulation.

Structural reflex zone therapy for labour

5

INTRODUCTION

Intrapartum reflex zone therapy (RZT) can be a valuable aid to progress and comfort, but should normally only be given by midwives or by experienced therapists with a thorough understanding of the dynamic nature of labour and birth, and a sophisticated ability to relate theory to practice. Therapists who are not qualified midwives should always defer to the midwife responsible for the mother's care and discuss with her whether it is appropriate to provide therapy or, later, to continue. Therapists intending to accompany women in labour should seek permission to do so from the midwife *before* the onset of labour, even if the mother is having a home birth, and should ensure that their indemnity insurance covers them to provide reflexology during labour and birth.

Unlike treatment during the antenatal period, RZT in labour may be given in short intermittent treatments over several hours, according to the mother's wishes and maternal and fetal wellbeing. The practitioner may need to adapt the treatment to fit in with the mother's contractions and progress. Not all women want to be touched during contractions; indeed, some women who have planned to receive reflexology in labour may change their minds at the last moment and the independent practitioner should be aware of this, as her role may need to change to being more of a labour supporter than a reflexologist. One of the principal benefits of RZT is that it requires the attendance of the practitioner – and this in itself can be immensely comforting to the mother and to the practitioner, in a return to the traditional role of being "with woman". This can be particularly pertinent in busy maternity units where a mother may not have her midwife in the room with her for the entire duration of the labour.

As with normal maternity notes, records should be maintained contemporaneously, because the maternal or fetal condition can change suddenly and it may be difficult to remember accurately precisely what occurred if note-writing is left until later. A record should be made of the justification for performing RZT, the time of commencing and ending treatment. This record should be in the normal maternity notes (if performed by a midwife), in the therapist's own notes (if performed by an independent practitioner) and on the cardiotocograph paper if the mother is being electronically monitored (although this may be considered a contraindication to RZT in some units).

The practitioner should be very clear about the indications for performing RZT during labour and should take care not to overstep professional boundaries. Treatment should start only with very gentle relaxation stroking, *extremely* light sedation to the "solar plexus" zone and plenty of holding movements in order to accustom the mother to the treatment at such a dynamic psychological and physiological time, and for the practitioner to assess the mother's reactions. The pressure and type of treatment techniques used can be built up as appropriate, but women may experience reactions very quickly in labour and care should be taken to avoid this. In particular, "solar plexus" sedation applied at too deep a pressure or maintained for too long can cause restlessness, breathlessness, nausea and palpitations: if this occurs it may be necessary to apply light sedation to the adrenal gland zones for 3–5 seconds and then to stimulate (i.e. massage *gently*) the "solar plexus". On the other hand, some apparently adverse reactions may not be in response to the RZT, but may be a feature of the mother's labour, or could be the onset of deviations from the norm. This fact emphasises the need for a thorough appreciation of labour physiology and maternal behaviour.

PAIN RELIEF IN LABOUR

Structural physiology and aetiology

There is a growing body of evidence to demonstrate that touch and therapies involving manual contact act as a pain-relieving strategy, since touch impulses reach the brain before pain impulses and the impact of endorphin release aids this (Garner et al 2008, Kimber et al 2008, Mitchinson et al 2007, Seers et al 2008). It has also been demonstrated that anxiety and cortisol levels may be reduced, specifically with reflexology (McVicar et al 2007). RZT treatment of mothers in labour should be both general (relaxation) and aimed at relieving pain in the relevant areas of the body, as they experience labour pain in many different ways. It is useful to remember that, whilst pain is a normal component of labour, the mother may need some help to cope with the intensity of the contractions, particularly as the first stage progresses.

Normal progress in labour depends on the interaction of the uterine contractions, fetal position and descent and the shape of the bony pelvis. Uterine contractions are triggered hormonally by the release of oxytocin in the pituitary gland, which contracts smooth muscle; the continual contraction of the muscle fibres then causes pain. The body's natural reaction to pain is to produce endorphins to subdue the sensation. However, fear, anxiety and the anticipation of pain may cause premature release of endorphins in an attempt to overcome these emotions, which in turn inhibits the release of oxytocin. The contractions do not then become efficient enough to trigger sufficient beneficial release of endorphins and a negative cycle of events occurs in which the mother experiences pain but the contractions remain inefficient. Furthermore, the rise in stress hormones such as cortisol and adrenaline (epinephrine) may also inhibit the action of oxytocin – so the relaxation effect of reflexology is hugely positive in ensuring homeostasis at this time.

Mechanically, the contractions commence from the pacemakers situated in the junction where the fallopian tube enters the uterine fundus, leading to fundal/abdominal pain. Neurological pain pathways in the first stage are related to the spine segments at the level of the first and second lumbar vertebrae, the lower abdomen and the groin area, from the sympathetic nerves from the uterus. Tension on the uterosacral ligaments causes lumbosacral backache, commonly much worse when the fetal position is posterior, which can only be relieved when the angle of the pelvic brim alters, tipping forwards. Although most women experience pain in the abdominal, suprapubic, lumbosacral and inner thigh areas, some may also complain of pain further down the legs, as well as shoulder and neck pain, which may be exacerbated by the mother's emotional state and by her position.

In the second stage, pain becomes focused more in the perineal area and is mediated through the sacral nerve plexus at the level of the second to fourth sacral vertebrae. Downwards pressure of the diaphragm aids fetal descent, whereas the pelvic floor muscles relax to accommodate the descending fetus and to facilitate rotation to the most favourable position for birth (occipito anterior). Somatic pain in the second stage is felt in the vagina, rectum, anus, perineal area and inner thighs. Changes also occur within the bony pelvis as the fetus descends and rotates, particularly in the late first and the second stage. These adaptations include flexion of the lumbosacral joint, backwards movement of the sacrum (counternutation), sacroiliac joint torsion, stretching of the symphysis pubis and pubic arch and/or flexion of the sacrococcygeal joint, depending on whether the fetal position is anterior or posterior (Stone 2007:315).

Relevant reflexology treatment

RZT is especially useful in labour for its relaxation effect and treatment should include frequent, repeated stroking, holding and diaphragm "sweeping". A sustained sedation of the "solar plexus" zones can be applied both during and between contractions, for up to 2 minutes at a time (Lett 2000:227), although this should be very gentle at first with no indentation of the skin until the practitioner has ascertained that the mother can tolerate a deeper pressure. Either of these techniques can be used with the mother in any position, including sitting on a birthing ball, on all fours, sitting or lying in a semi-recumbent or lateral position, but the practitioner should be alert to her own posture and comfort as well as that of the mother. If the mother is mobile,

Structural reflex zone therapy for labour

her hands can be treated with firm even stroking and "solar plexus" sedation. These techniques are also helpful prior to or during vaginal examination or if an epidural cannula is being inserted.

If the mother is on a bed or sitting in a chair and there is time for a longer treatment, this may include:

- diaphragm "sweeping" and "caterpillar crawling" over the lung zones to ease the diaphragm and regulate breathing
- stimulation (massage) of the zones for the scapulae to release toxins accumulated through shoulder tension
- cupping the heels in the hands, with the "heels" of the practitioner's hands on the mother's outer heels and the length of the fingers placed over the inner heels (taking care not to press inadvertently with the fingertips), applied either as a sustained pressure for the duration of each contraction or intermittently, depending on the mother's preference. This is calming and analgesic and effectively applies a diversified pressure over the zones for the reproductive organs
- manipulation of the zones for the whole spine, plus sedation of the zones for the first to second lumbar (or second to fourth sacral vertebrae if the second stage appears imminent)
- manipulation of the ankles to aid changes within the bony pelvis
- sedating techniques on the zones for the sacroiliac joints, especially if the mother is experiencing lower backache
- general "caterpillar crawling" as with a full-length relaxation treatment for no longer than 20–30 minutes, although practitioners should be prepared to pause or discontinue treatment at any time depending on the mother's progress and the need for any midwifery observations or care
- sweeping movements across the area of the ankle corresponding to the fallopian tubes and the pelvic lymphatics can ease pelvic congestion; however, a more effective technique is to ask the mother to massage her own wrists in a "Chinese burn" movement, over the hand reflex zone for her pelvic lymphatics. She can perform this periodically throughout the labour, first on one wrist and then the other.

ESTIMATION OF THE ONSET OF LABOUR WITH REFLEX ZONE THERAPY

This author has used a reflex zone diagnostic technique for many years to determine whether a mother's labour is imminent. Although the technique has not been formally evaluated, other colleagues are now using the system successfully, particularly in relation to the potential success of medical induction. The technique requires the practitioner to be able to identify accurately the precise point for the (indirect) reflex zone for the pituitary gland (as used in this book, see Chapter 3 and Fig. 3.1a). Each pituitary reflex zone is then pressed in turn, starting with the point on the right foot, and the mother is asked to grade, on a scale of 1–10, the intensity of tenderness felt (1 = no pain, 10 = extremely painful). Care should be taken that the amount of pressure applied and the number of presses are equal on both sides as continued pressure increases the tenderness.

Accumulated experience appears to suggest that the pituitary point on the right foot is tender throughout pregnancy, inferring that it is consistent with ongoing antenatal pituitary activity. However, the pituitary point on the left foot appears to become increasingly tender as pregnancy progresses, perhaps reflecting the upheaval in hormonal activity towards term as pregnancy hormones decline and, correspondingly, labour hormone levels increase. When the pituitary zone on the mother's left foot is more tender than that on the right, this appears to suggest that labour is imminent, albeit based on a subjective assessment by the mother on the severity of tenderness. (A key to remembering this system is to think "left = labour".)

This system can be helpful – and encouraging – to mothers. It is not possible, at this stage, to be precise about the onset of labour, although a "guesstimate" can be made by this author to within 1–2 days. Anecdotal evidence does, however, appear to correlate this pituitary zone tenderness with the success or otherwise of medical induction of labour (prostin, amniotomy or syntocinon). In short, induction appears to be more likely to proceed well and the mother's labour to become properly established if the pituitary zone on the left foot is more tender than that on the right. Conversely, if the right pituitary zone is more tender than that on the left, induction appears more likely to result in complications, a cascade of intervention and the possibility of Caesarean section. (See also Chapter 3 regarding prediction of the menstrual cycle in non-pregnant women.)

INDUCTION AND ACCELERATION OF LABOUR

Structural physiology and aetiology

It cannot be stressed strongly enough that *induction of labour* is a medical procedure for a specified medical or obstetric indication and it is not within the realm of the reflexologist's responsibility to attempt to induce labour before the mother's due date. However, there are occasions when the mother does not commence labour spontaneously and is offered medical induction, usually after a prescribed period of 10–14 days past the due date, depending on the policies of the local obstetricians. Many women dislike the idea of being subjected to something that is a medical intervention in a natural process and fear the loss of control that this engenders. It is interesting to note that mothers – and many midwifery and reflexology professionals – fail to appreciate that using RZT to stimulate contractions could also be viewed as an intervention in the physiological process of childbirth, despite the fact that it is "natural".

Research has, however, shown that receiving regular reflexology towards the end of pregnancy contributes to spontaneous onset of labour, improves progress and outcome, and reduces maternal pain perception (Feder et al 1994, Motha & McGrath 1993). This early research, specifically on reflexology, has not been replicated but more contemporary studies on touch and massage in general indicate similar effects on labour (Field et al 2008a). General relaxation treatment may thus be sufficient to facilitate this process, especially as the balance between oxytocin, stress hormones and endorphins can be restored to equilibrium. However, when a decision is made that specific RZT techniques are justified to try to induce labour this should be performed only by a midwife or by an experienced reflexologist who has discussed the individual mother's case with the midwife and who understands the relevant physiology and potential pathology.

Failure to progress – requiring acceleration of contractions after labour is deemed to have commenced – occurs for a variety of reasons and it is essential for reflexologists who are not midwives to confer with the midwife responsible for the mother's care as to whether it is safe to use reflexology techniques to assist in this process. Most causes of slow labour are related to the inter-relationship between the powers (contractions), the passages (pelvis and cervix) and the passenger (fetus). When a mother has been in established labour, which later slows down, it may be because she is tired or dehydrated and lacks the energy for her body to produce effective uterine contractions. This can be rectified relatively easily and contractions may either recommence spontaneously or can be stimulated with oxytocic drugs or with RZT. More seriously, there may be disproportion between the size and shape of the bony pelvis and the size and position of the fetus. In late first stage there may be just an anterior "lip" of cervix remaining before full dilatation of the cervix is achieved, which can cause distress for the mother and a prolonged transition stage. The potential cause *must* be determined *before* attempting to use RZT to accelerate labour, especially in a multigravida, because over-stimulating contractions, by any means, when labour has become obstructed may precipitate serious complications including – in extreme (but rare) circumstances – uterine rupture, profuse haemorrhage or fetal – or even maternal – death.

An interesting phenomenon which may assist in identifying when a mother's labour is beginning to deviate from normal has been observed by midwives working with this author. It appears that the outer heels of women whose labour is failing to progress take on a reddish, mottled appearance, perhaps suggesting congestion in the reflex zones for the pelvic organs. These changes in the heels are seen to occur prior to the clinical diagnosis of "failure to progress", and the finding is now being used informally as an aid to diagnosis, although no structured clinical trials have yet been undertaken.

It is not appropriate for reflexologists to attempt to induce or accelerate labour without first discussing it with the midwife responsible for the mother's care to determine whether or not it is safe to do so, based on the individual mother's circumstances.

Relevant reflexology treatment

It has already been stated that labour contractions are influenced by the release of oxytocin from the pituitary gland, therefore it would be incorrect to stimulate the reflex zone for the uterus; indeed, this could potentially interfere with the process of labour and theoretically result in complications, such as placental separation and haemorrhage. The effect of fear and pain on oxytocin production has also been discussed, and if the pregnancy is post dates and the mother is being "threatened" with medical induction she may become very anxious and agitated. General relaxation reflexology may be enough, therefore, to calm her and encourage eutocic action. In any situation where there is doubt about whether or not it is appropriate to use RZT to induce labour, the relaxation techniques should be used first and the practitioner should then wait to evaluate their outcome.

Specific RZT treatment involves stimulation of the two pituitary gland zones on the big toes, usually working on one then the other, rather than both together which can be too strong and which may initiate hypertonic uterine action. Intermittent stimulation of up to thirty presses can be applied, although it may be necessary to stop before this number is reached as the mother may find it too uncomfortable. If a general treatment is being given, pituitary stimulation can be repeated periodically throughout the relaxation session – this may be more effective and cause less acute discomfort to the mother.

It is not the purpose of this book to include other complementary therapies which may be useful when caring for pregnant and childbearing clients (see Further reading). However, there are several acupressure points on the feet and legs which can be effective for induction/acceleration of labour and which can easily be incorporated into a foot treatment which comprises primarily RZT, with or without foot massage. It is paramount, however, that the practitioner using these additional strategies is *absolutely clear* whether she is performing RZT or acupressure. From a clinical perspective the mother will simply receive a treatment in which pressure is applied to the feet, but from a professional perspective the practitioner must be able to define precisely the treatment that is being given. Furthermore, she must be able to support and justify her actions with reference to relevant research findings.

Acupuncture/acupressure is based on the notion that the body has energy lines (meridians) running through it which carry the body's life force (*qi*, pronounced *chee*) and which link one part of the body to others. These meridians each pass through a major organ of the body, after which the energy line is named. There are 14 major and 365 minor meridians in a branching network throughout the body, including the Heart, Gall Bladder, Spleen, Stomach, Liver meridians, etc. Each meridian has a number of focus points (acupoints or *tsubos*) along it, numbered from 1 to a variable number, depending on the length of the meridian; they are thought to be similar to, or linked to, anatomical trigger points (Baldry 2005). In optimum health, the individual's life force flows around the body unhindered, but physical, mental or spiritual distress or disease causes blockages or excesses of energy at certain acupoints along the meridians. Rebalancing of the body's energy involves stimulation or sedation of the relevant points, which can be achieved through the application of thumb pressure (acupressure), insertion of needles (acupuncture) or with other methods such as cupping (sedation) and moxibustion (stimulation). Stimulation of some acupoints is contraindicated during pregnancy as they are known to initiate contractions and could potentially trigger preterm labour, but at term they can legitimately be used to facilitate progress.

There is considerable research evidence to support the use of specific acupressure points to stimulate contractions, including Spleen 6, usually together with points on the shoulders (Gall Bladder 21) and on the hands (Large Intestine 4) (Gaudernack et al 2006, Ingram et al 2005). Stimulation applied to these acupoints repeated on alternate days from the due date, has been shown to facilitate cervical ripening and reduce the interval between the expected date of delivery and spontaneous onset of labour (Rabl et al 2001), although systematic reviews by Smith et al (2008) and Selmer-Olsen et al (2007) refuted these claims. Various other studies have shown shorter first stages, fewer Caesarean sections and greater pain relief following acupressure, than in controls (Chang et al 2004, Gaudet et al 2008, Harper et al 2006, Lee et al 2004). Although there are acupoints elsewhere on the body which may help in this process, these are not discussed here, and the only points to be used in conjunction with structural RZT are found on the feet and legs, namely Spleen 6, Bladder 60 and Bladder 67.

Spleen 6 is the most potent of the points for stimulating contractions. The Spleen meridian starts on the corner of the toe nail on the medial aspect of each big toe and runs up the inner aspect of each leg. It passes through the inguinal region, up the abdominal and thoracic areas, lateral to the midline, around the distal edge of the breast to the second intercostal space and then descends past the axilla to the level of the eleventh rib. The Spleen 6 acupoint is located three Chinese inches (*cun*), or approximately three finger widths, above the medial malleolus (inner ankle bone), on the posterior border of the tibia (on both legs). Spleen 6 (or Sanyinjiao) is said to be useful (in non-pregnant clients) for tiredness, loss of appetite, diarrhoea, urinary conditions, for calming the mind, tonifying the kidneys and rebalancing Liver meridian energy, and for a variety of gynaecological disorders. Stimulation to Spleen 6 is normally contraindicated in pregnancy until term. The point will be painful when pressure is applied; indeed, women often report that the point throbs for the rest of the day when they have had stimulation to facilitate the onset of labour (see Fig. 5.1). The point should be stimulated by pressing

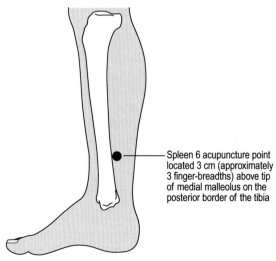

Spleen 6 acupuncture point located 3 cm (approximately 3 finger-breadths) above tip of medial malleolus on the posterior border of the tibia

Fig. 5.1   Spleen 6 acupuncture point

firmly with the thumbs, intermittently for up to thirty presses or for as long as the mother can tolerate it, if this is less. It is wise to work on the Spleen 6 point on both legs simultaneously as the mother may find it too uncomfortable if they are stimulated separately. This is the most dynamic of the points for induction and acceleration and can sometimes have an almost immediate effect. It can be useful when the fetal head remains high above the pelvic brim as good uterine contractions will cause flexion of the fetal head allowing it to descend. However, the reflexologist who is not a midwife will need to discuss with the midwife to determine if it is appropriate to perform this technique.

Both the Bladder 60 and Bladder 67 acupoints are powerful points which stimulate downwards movement from the uterus. The Bladder 67 point is difficult to palpate manually; it is more normally stimulated with acupuncture needles or with moxibustion for women with a breech presentation (i.e. promoting downwards movement of the fetal head, see Chapter 4), but it is not the most accessible for induction or acceleration of labour. On the other hand, the Bladder 60 acupoint is very effective at encouraging downwards movement of the fetal presenting part, or of the placenta on some occasions when there is delay in the second stage (see below). However, due to the complex aetiology when a mother's labour fails to progress at the anticipated rate, these acupoints should only be used by experienced practitioners who are trained to use RZT with acupressure and who can apply theory to practice. Enthusiastic and well-meaning stimulation of the Bladder 60 point by a practitioner who has not rationalised the pathophysiological processes can cause impaction of the presenting part. For example, if the fetal head is not well flexed the biparietal diameter may become trapped in the sacrocotyloid diameter of the posterior pelvis, leading to possible extension of the fetal neck and a complicated brow presentation, which is usually not compatible with vaginal delivery. In order for the head to flex adequately to move downwards in the pelvis, the uterus must first contract efficiently. It is of immense concern that at least one textbook known to this author, intended for midwives learning reflexology, encourages "strong stimulation" of both Bladder 60 and 67 "to expedite labour", but does not qualify this statement with the relevant safety issues. If there is any doubt regarding flexion of the presenting part it is more appropriate to stimulate the reflex zone for the pituitary gland or the Spleen 6 acupoint. If, however, the midwife is confident that the head is well flexed but still relatively high in the pelvic cavity, stimulation of the Bladder 60 acupoint, with intermittent pressure can be effective at encouraging descent in the first or early second stage of labour.

The Bladder meridian is a long line, commencing in the inner corner of each eye, travelling up over the top of the head to the occipital ridge. Here, it divides, with one line running down the back from the neck, along the inner edge of the scapula to the lumbar region. The other line runs straight down the middle of the back to the lumbar area and then descends down the back of the leg; eventually curling around the outer ankle bone and ending in the outer edge at the base of the little toe nail (Bladder 67 acupoint). The Bladder 60 (or Kunlun) point is located in a depression between the tip of the lateral (outer) malleolus and the Achilles tendon (see Fig. 5.2).

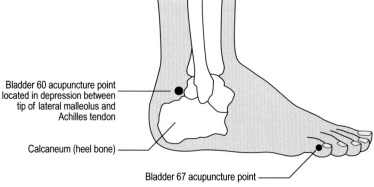

Bladder 60 acupuncture point located in depression between tip of lateral malleolus and Achilles tendon

Calcaneum (heel bone)

Bladder 67 acupuncture point

Fig. 5.2 Bladder 60 and Bladder 67 acupuncture points

CASE STUDY 5.1 INDUCTION OF LABOUR

Geraldine and her partner visited the midwife-reflexologist's antenatal clinic when Geraldine was 41 weeks pregnant with her first baby. She was booked for medical induction of labour 5 days later, but was anxious to go into labour spontaneously as she wanted to have a home water birth and she had not yet had any of the signs of impending labour. Although Geraldine used several complementary therapies at home, her partner was sceptical about using points on the feet to trigger contractions and was concerned about the wellbeing of Geraldine and the baby. The nature of the clinic did not allow time for long relaxation sessions and it was explained that, if they agreed, treatment would consist only of stimulation of various points with the specific aim of starting labour.

The midwife started the manual session by palpating the reflex zones for the pituitary gland and found that the reflex zone on Geraldine's left foot was extremely tender – Geraldine assessed it as being 10/10 – whereas the point on her right foot was estimated at 4/10. This suggested that Geraldine's labour was imminent and that any reflex zone therapy (RZT) treatment would serve to expedite the onset. The midwife stimulated the two reflex zones for the pituitary gland and the Spleen 6 acupressure point above the inner ankles, which were also immensely tender. This had the immediate effect of causing the uterus to harden with a mild contraction each time the points were stimulated. The hands-on treatment lasted about 15 minutes and the appointment lasted another 10 minutes whilst the midwife completed the notes and answered a few more questions. However, during this time Geraldine had two distinct uterine contractions, which were significantly more painful than the normal Braxton Hicks contractions of pregnancy, and was complaining of backache and suprapubic pain as she left the clinic; her husband was very surprised and confessed to "being converted"! Three hours later they returned to the delivery suite and after another 4 hours Geraldine gave birth to a lovely baby girl.

> Reflexologists should not assume that a labour in which the fetal presenting part remains high can be automatically treated with stimulation of the Bladder 60 acupressure point to encourage descent. It is *vital* to determine first whether there is any cephalopelvic disproportion, as injudicious stimulation of Bladder 60 can precipitate major complications, such as obstructed labour and, in extreme cases, uterine rupture, torrential haemorrhage and fetal or even maternal mortality.

RETAINED PLACENTA

Structural physiology and aetiology

The third stage of labour is the most hazardous for the mother and a mismanaged third stage can be fatal due to torrential haemorrhage. Therapists who are not midwives *must* discuss with the midwife to determine if it is safe or appropriate to use RZT to expedite the placental delivery. They must also understand fully the relevant physiopathology of the individual mother. The length of the third stage of labour will depend on whether it is managed physiologically or actively by the midwife. A natural third stage may last between 20 and 60 minutes, whereas a third stage for which the mother has received oxytocic medication is usually completed within 5 to 20 minutes, although there are fairly wide variations. If the third stage becomes prolonged (after about an hour) the most common reason is that the placenta has not yet separated; alternatively it may have separated and have not been expelled, perhaps being trapped behind the cervix or lying in the vagina.

Midwifery management of a retained placenta is dictated by whether the mother is bleeding and whether the uterus is well contracted. If the uterus is not well contracted there will be heavier vaginal bleeding than expected and this can rapidly lead to maternal collapse, if not attended to; the urgency of the situation is in direct correlation to the amount of blood loss and the reason for the haemorrhage. Other causes of bleeding include lacerations in the vagina or cervix, a full bladder preventing adequate uterine contraction or haematological conditions, such as severe anaemia or clotting disorders. If the mother is bleeding profusely it is entirely inappropriate for her to be treated with RZT.

Relevant reflexology treatment

Using RZT to treat a mother with a retained placenta is an example of how the therapy can be used as a "first aid" tool, in a way which may be criticised by some as being reductionist. However, mismanagement can precipitate major complications such as haemorrhage and it is essential to determine the extent to which RZT can be administered – and when it is appropriate to turn to conventional pharmacological and/or surgical management. It is not usually appropriate, nor is there normally enough time, to incorporate many of the general relaxation techniques used in antenatal and first stage treatments. Furthermore, in the case of an independent therapist accompanying a mother in labour, it is vital that she communicates with the midwife responsible for the mother's care, to ensure that both understand the aim of the RZT treatment.

If the uterus is not well contracted the priority is to encourage it to do so and the decision as to whether an attempt can be made to facilitate this with RZT or whether it is more appropriate to administer drugs must be made by the midwife. If it is felt that it may be worthwhile to try RZT, the pituitary gland zones should be stimulated intermittently for 20–30 presses and then repeated according to the mother's tolerance and progress. This may, of course, be combined with putting the baby to the breast to suckle in an attempt to stimulate natural oxytocin, or even used alongside the administration of oxytocic drugs. Sometimes this is sufficient to encourage the placenta to contract; the placenta will then separate and descend, and can be delivered either by the mother pushing it out or by the midwife applying controlled cord traction. This treatment can also be used when the mother is experiencing moderate bleeding, even when the placenta has been expelled, but should not be attempted if haemorrhage is severe. In the event that the third stage of labour has become so prolonged that the mother is advised to have a manual removal of the placenta, it may be worthwhile continuing the relevant treatment whilst awaiting the anaesthetic: several cases are known to this author in which repeated stimulation of the pituitary gland zones has resolved the problem at the last minute in the anaesthetic room. This attempt to encourage the uterus to contract can also be aided by stimulation of the Spleen 6 acupoint.

If the uterus is already well contracted there is no real indication to stimulate the pituitary gland zones, especially if oxytocic drugs have already been administered. Indeed, continued stimulation may cause the cervix to clamp down, trapping the partially or wholly separated placenta behind it and effectively preventing the uterus from remaining well contracted, potentially leading to haemorrhage. It is now necessary for the midwife to identify the possible cause of the retained placenta before proceeding with RZT or any other strategies. If the placenta has separated and the uterus remains well contracted with minimal bleeding, the practitioner can encourage descent by stimulation of the Bladder 60 acupressure point on both legs.

CASE STUDY 5.2   RETAINED PLACENTA

Robyn, a gravida 3, para 2, had arrived in the delivery suite in established labour and delivered one hour after being admitted, having been knowingly contracting for only 4 hours. The birth of the baby was also rapid and the second stage was completed in 10 minutes. Despite being given an oxytocic drug as the baby was born, the placenta did not appear to have separated after 50 minutes, although the uterus was well contracted and there was no undue blood loss. Another dose of oxytocin was administered, but the placenta still did not separate, and after another 40 minutes had passed it was decided by the obstetric registrar that Robyn needed a manual removal of the placenta under general anaesthetic.

CASE STUDY 5.2   RETAINED PLACENTA—CONT'D

Robyn was moved to the theatre, but by chance the midwife there was approved to use reflex zone therapy (RZT). She stimulated the reflex zones for the pituitary, although Robyn found this extremely uncomfortable, together with the Spleen 6 acupoint, followed by stimulation of the Bladder 60 acupressure point, which appeared to cause a lengthening of the umbilical cord emerging from the vagina and an intense contraction of the uterus. Whether this treatment had caused the placenta to separate or not is difficult to say, but it may have provided a final stimulation to encourage normal physiology to proceed. Fortunately, Robyn did not need to have the manual removal, for which she was immensely grateful.

Structural reflex zone therapy for labour

Structural reflex zone therapy for the puerperium

INTRODUCTION

Reflex zone therapy (RZT) can be an invaluable tool for assisting new mothers with recovery from pregnancy and birth and for enhancing wellbeing at this time of immense psycho-social and hormonal upheaval as they adapt to their new roles. If the mother has had a normal birth she could be offered RZT treatments daily during the immediate post-delivery week to aid a return to homeostasis, but obviously this is dependent on time and staffing constraints and is not usually a feasible option unless the mother requests an independent reflexologist to visit her, either in hospital or at home. After the first week, if the mother has access to an independent therapist, treatment can be given twice weekly, then weekly until the end of the puerperium. As with the antenatal period, RZT offers the mother valuable "me time" and a respite from the perpetual round of caring for the new baby, however enjoyable that may be.

If the mother has had an instrumental or operative delivery, daily treatments are not appropriate, because her body needs more time to recover from the pathological consequences of the delivery, and reactions to treatment may mask iatrogenic complications. A treatment every 2 to 3 days is acceptable in the first 2 weeks, then twice weekly for a few weeks, then weekly for as long as the mother wishes.

In addition, reflexology can be wonderful for the baby, either performed by the practitioner or by teaching the parents some basic techniques which can be used to keep the baby calm and to aid adaptation to extra-uterine life. There is a considerable body of evidence on the beneficial effects of touch with regard to newborn infants; it has been shown to increase growth and body weight in those born preterm (Chen et al 2008), to influence perinatal programming for health in adulthood (Hodgson et al 2007) and to reduce the incidence of postnatal depression when used by mothers to massage their babies (Fujita et al 2006, O'Higgins et al 2008). However, it is not the intention of this book to explore specific RZT treatments for the neonate, and readers are referred to Marquardt (2000:194–199) and Lett (2000:233–241) for more information.

Most mothers, who have given birth in a hospital setting, will be transferred home within 24 hours of delivery; those with complications or who have had an operative delivery may stay in hospital for a few days. British midwifery has always prided itself on providing comprehensive postnatal care for the mother and baby, which was hitherto unlike any other postnatal care in the world, with the exception of the Netherlands. However, reductions in staffing and a change in priorities have led to a vast reduction in routine postnatal care, with the number of home visits by a midwife limited in many areas to three, although some maternity services offer a postnatal "drop in" facility. While this appears to satisfy the majority of mothers insofar as their physical wellbeing is concerned, many would benefit from more overt moral support from their midwives with regard to their psychological wellbeing and also for assistance with establishment of breast feeding. Furthermore, a change in the focus of postnatal care from a monitoring of the mother's physical needs to facilitation of the psycho-social aspects of early parenthood could contribute to better breast-feeding rates, and greater maternal – and midwifery – satisfaction.

Reflexology practitioners who are midwives often report that pregnant and postnatal women reveal far more information during an RZT treatment session than during a conventional antenatal appointment or postnatal examination, asking more questions and expressing more concerns than they might otherwise have done. Thus, RZT/reflexology could, perhaps controversially, present a new means of providing postnatal care in the 21st century. Offering a 15 minute session of relaxation RZT instead of focusing on the physiopathological changes such as involution, lochial discharges and perineal healing, would give the mother a sense of being nurtured, could alter her perception of the discomforts of the puerperium and provide her with the opportunity to ask questions. This would be especially beneficial as a means of de-briefing the mother following delivery and would enable her to rest and relax. The midwife would be alert to possible physiological and psychological deviations from the norm, perhaps identifying early breast-feeding difficulties or abnormal fluctuations in the mother's mood and then being able to rectify them before they develop into more severe complications. Practitioners who are not midwives could report to the midwife with any issues that are outside the parameters of normality; these non-midwife practitioners could be either fully qualified reflexologists or maternity support workers who have been trained to perform simple relaxation reflexology techniques.

PSYCHO-EMOTIONAL RECOVERY FROM BIRTH

Structural physiology and aetiology

For the majority of mothers, the arrival of the new baby is a joyous event. Initially the mother will be on a "high", but this is often followed by a sense of anticlimax as the adrenaline (epinephrine) levels subside after delivery and she begins to realise the enormity of the event and the responsibilities with which she is now faced. Added to this, the expulsion of the placenta eliminates the remaining source of pregnancy hormones, which causes plummeting levels of oestrogen, progesterone, etc. In response, the lactation hormones are released, leading to further hormonal upheaval and emotional lability – the "baby blues" – which occurs at about 3–4 days after the birth. Most new mothers also feel physically uncomfortable immediately after the birth, even when they have had a straightforward labour and delivery. The mother may have specific pain from the delivery, or more generalised aches and weariness. Later, as the milk supply increases, the mother can suffer breast discomfort and soreness.

Tiredness is a real issue for most new mothers who have their sleep patterns disrupted nightly. This may be exacerbated by pain and discomfort, and by anxieties about the baby's wellbeing, establishing feeding and practical issues related to baby care, as well as social and domestic problems which may be present, such as returning to work, and financial or relationship difficulties. Excitement may make it difficult for the mother to sleep even when she has time and opportunity, or she may wake up spontaneously in the night, especially if her breasts are full.

Mothers who have had any intervention during the labour will feel particularly uncomfortable; they may have headache, back, leg and neck pain following epidural anaesthesia, perineal pain from an episiotomy or excessive tearing, severe vaginal and vulval pain after a forceps delivery or ongoing abdominal pain if they have had a Caesarean section. RZT can be extremely beneficial for these mothers in helping them to recover emotionally, as well as physically, as they often have a feeling of "grief" at not having achieved a normal delivery; this may also be extended to mothers who have had an induction of labour. Similarly, mothers whose babies are ill and have been admitted to the special or intensive care baby unit, or even a mother whose baby has died, may find solace in having regular RZT treatments in the early weeks after delivery. However, it is important that the practitioner has a thorough understanding of the nature of the baby's complications or the reason for the baby's death, as well as well-refined listening skills, because the mother may welcome the sessions as an opportunity for emotional release, or she may require specific medical details of her case.

Psychological stress and tension lead to physical (structural or mechanical) manifestations which overload the body's general adaptive response and adversely affect the immune system. People who are stressed often habitually hold the muscles of the head, neck or lower back in a state of tension, eventually leading to pain. Further, anxiety and stress impair the functioning of the limbic system, which in turn also causes spasm in the muscles of the neck, because they contain a higher proportion of afferent fibres than most other striated muscles, making them more sensitive; this is thought to be one of the reasons why tension headaches occur with stress (Middleditch & Oliver 2005:103). Spasm of the muscles in the occiput, where some of the neck muscles are attached, is caused by tension on the periosteum, while contraction of the muscles of the cervical vertebrae causes referred pain in the temporomandibular joint of the face and in the jaw. Tension on the sternocleidomastoid and trapezius muscles, often brought about by compensatory adjustments to the angle of the head in an attempt to subdue the neck pain, may then lead to shoulder pain. Psychological and emotional stress affects the sympathetic nervous system which, therefore, influences pain perception through neuochemical changes. In mothers undergoing long-term stress with physical effects, pain occurs due to the accumulation of metabolites in the muscles, which are a source of irritation; this perpetuates the muscular contraction and leads to a vicious cycle, which, if unchecked, can result in restriction in the joints and loss of mobility.

Whilst some stress and anxiety, together with "baby blues"in the early days, is normal, a few mothers develop more serious psychiatric disorders, such as postnatal depression or psychosis, in the weeks and months following the birth. Others experience a form of post-traumatic stress disorder, most commonly when there have been serious complications in labour, perhaps with emergency measures needing to be implemented, or where the baby is ill or has died. In some women these conditions may last up to a year, and in a few, may herald the onset of chronic depression or precipitate the development of latent bipolar disorder. Although no formal evidence of a musculoskeletal link to postnatal depression could be found when searching the contemporary literature, osteopaths theorise that a mechanically difficult labour may compress the sacrum between the lateral borders of the bones of the pelvis, particularly the ilia, leading to neurogenic compromise along the length of the spine to the brain, triggering neurological pathology (personal communication with osteopathy tutor).

Relevant reflexology treatment

It is neither realistic nor practical to differentiate between the physical and the psychological factors inherent in the puerperium, as one affects the other. Therefore, treatment in the early postnatal period should aim to nurture the mother and aid her recovery from birth by easing pain and discomfort and facilitating her ability to cope with the physical and emotional changes she is experiencing. Relaxation reflexology treatments may also help the mother to rest when she is very tired, possibly inducing sleep; it is, therefore, wise to discuss the timing of the treatment so that she can arrange for someone to look after the baby.

Structural reflex zone therapy for the puerperium

A whole relaxation treatment can be performed to aid the return to non-pregnant homeostasis, to ease muscular and psychological fatigue and to balance the whole system. However, care should be taken not to over-stimulate any specific reflex zones unless appropriate, as her reactions to RZT treatment may be rapid and profound, especially in the first 24 hours after delivery. Specific RZT techniques should only be performed when there is an indication to do so, but it is useful to include plenty of calming and relaxing movements in the regular relaxation treatments to aid normal physiology:

- gentle "solar plexus" work to relax the mother
- *stimulation* of the adrenal zones if she has a post-adrenaline "slump" immediately after the birth *or gentle sedation* of the adrenal gland reflex zones if she shows signs of remaining hyper-stimulated immediately after delivery – however, no direct adrenal zone work should be performed later unless there is a strong adrenaline surge for some reason
- "diaphragm sweeping" and stimulating movements over the lung reflex zones to regulate breathing and help re-establish respiration from the bases of the lungs which have been compressed in late pregnancy
- working over the reflex zones for the endocrine system in order to tone and regulate; this should be neither stimulation nor sedation, but "caterpillar crawling" across the zones
- gentle working of the reflex zones for the head, neck, spine, pelvis to release tension
- specifically working along the renal tract zones with the "caterpillar walking" technique to facilitate kidney function and help in the excretion of excess fluid resulting from ischaemia and autolysis
- clockwise massage of the reflex zones for the intestines, to regulate the bowels and prevent constipation (NB care should be taken with women with insulin-dependent diabetes mellitus, as this can become temporarily more unstable in the first few days after delivery)
- drainage of all the lymphatic reflex zones, also to aid excretion of waste
- toning movements to stimulate the zones for the abdominal wall (with caution if there has been any divarification of the rectus sheath muscles, see below)
- stimulation and massage of the liver reflex zone is thought to assist detoxification when the mother has had large quanitites of drugs administered during labour or has had a Caesarean section.

Treatment should also include working on the reflex zones relevant to associated physical complaints, such as tension headaches, shoulder pain, perineal discomfort, etc.

Mothers suffering more profound emotional disturbances, postnatal depression and post-traumatic stress disorder may benefit from regular but short treatments to nurture them, aid sleep and calm them. However, it is essential to liaise with the medical team to ensure coordinated management of the mother's condition. Gentle manipulative techniques and stretching of the reflex zones for the spine, ribs and pelvis, as well as sedation of the sacroiliac joint and sciatic nerve reflex zones, may relieve sacral pressure and realign the pelvic bones, joints and ligaments. In cases where the mother has acute psychosis RZT is not appropriate, especially if she is taking antipsychotic drugs, as these may mask normal reactions to reflex zone treatment, or a combination of the two may complicate the overall clinical picture, causing difficulties for both conventional and complementary practitioners. Treatment should only be carried out by practitioners who are experienced in RZT, maternity care *and* who fully understand the psychiatric condition and its medical management. However, short treatments may be useful in combating the side effects of some of the drugs once the mother's reactions to them are known. It may be more acceptable to undertake a basic foot massage, incorporating only the very basic relaxation techniques, e.g. "solar plexus", diaphragm and lung reflex zones, with plenty of stroking and holding, rather than to work over the feet with "caterpillar crawling", while specific sedating or stimulating techniques should only be used with adequately rationalised justification.

MUSCULOSKELETAL SYSTEM

Structural physiology and aetiology

Backache in the postnatal period is common and is usually attributed to over-stretching of the transverse abdominus and other muscles, but may also be related to position during labour, the use of epidural anaesthesia or a pre-existing problem. Other musculoskeletal complaints may have developed during pregnancy but may persist for some while after delivery, including headache, carpal tunnel syndrome, sciatica, symphysis pubis diastasis or over-stretched abdominal muscles.

Postnatal tension and misalignment of the lower spine, occurring before pregnancy or as a result of antenatal hormonal changes and/or intrapartum events, places strain on the reproductive and abdominal organs and on the pelvic floor. This may be particularly significant if there has been excessive abduction of the legs in labour, since damage can occur in the joints and ligaments of the pelvis; pain occurs either as a result of direct muscle injury or as a reflex response to nociceptor irritation of joints and associated tissues: the use of the lithotomy position for forceps delivery, or the Trendelenburg position for Caesarean section, can cause activation of myofascial trigger points in the spine, leading to the development of chronic post-operative back pain (Baldry 2005:292). Poor abdominal muscle tone also contributes to ongoing back pain and associated problems in the longer term (Gustafsson & Nilsson-Wikmar 2008).

The increasing weight of the lactating breasts puts additional tension on the upper spine, head, neck and shoulder girdle, which further impacts on the lower musculoskeletal system. If the mother has a pre-existing lumbar problem which causes spasm in the erector spinae muscle she may complain of thoracic pain due to the attachment of the muscle to the ribs. Sometimes, pain will be felt in a referred area, for example, misalignment of the sacroiliac joint will cause spasm in the piriformis muscle, leading to discomfort in the buttocks and greater trochanters of the pelvis. Pain in the legs will be temporarily exacerbated if the mother adopts a posture in which she leans forwards. This is often observed on the postnatal ward in mothers who have had a Caesarean section; in order to compensate for the increased post-operative abdominal pain when walking, they lean forwards over the baby's cot for support, since the (new) discomfort felt in the legs is not as severe as the ongoing pain in the abdomen.

Misalignment of the spine can have a long-term impact on other internal organs and activate trigger points, which can cause other, seemingly unconnected symptoms and may impair the immune system. In this respect, the various ligaments play a major part in either supporting the organs or, if over-stretched, in causing alterations in the position of some organs, with consequent strain on others. The two broad ligaments, which support the uterus, are peritoneal structures continuous with the parietal peritoneum lining the abdominal walls and internal rectum. The peritoneum forms a mesenteric surface on which the lower gastrointestinal organs are able to slide and the broad ligaments basically form a floor to the abdominal cavity. The uterosacral and pubocervical ligaments support the lower one-third of the uterus and the vagina between the sacrum and the pubis; the transverse cervical (cardinal) ligaments stabilise the lower uterus and the cervix by attaching to the side walls of the pelvis. The uterosacral ligaments are inserted into the lower sacrum, coccyx, sacroiliac ligaments and piriformis muscle, and directly impact on the mechanics of the lumbar and sacral vertebrae and the hips. The round ligaments are continuous with the ovarian ligaments, passing from the uterine cornua through the inguinal canal, over the pubis and into the labia, anteriorly anchoring the uterus. In summary, the uterosacral ligaments influence the lower uterine segment and are related to sacral mechanics; the round ligaments provide lateral support, influencing the fundus and relating to the mechanics of the groin, symphysis pubis and perineum; the broad ligaments and fallopian tubes also influence the fundus and are related to the mechanics of the lateral abdomen, small intestines, sigmoid colon and caecum, near the appendix.

Thus it can be seen that dealing with back pain and other musculoskeletal problems is fundamental to the mother's overall recovery from pregnancy and delivery. Any factors which impact on the bony pelvis and lower spine will directly impact on the reproductive organs. Pre-conceptionally this may cause problems such as a retroverted uterus; antenatally, the disrupted relationship between the uterus and the pelvic brim may lead to malpresentation such as breech; and during labour a previous coccygeal fracture may not only reduce the pelvic outlet but also cause slight torsion on the uterus, potentially contributing to prolonged labour by adversely affecting the synergy between the upper and lower uterine segments. During the early puerperium, any of these factors may complicate her recovery, because the mother's body must overcome the impact of her personal musculoskeletal deviations in addition to those which are a part of normal physiological re-adaptation to the non-pregnant state; in addition, problems may persist in the long term, or develop as a consequence of poor management in the immediate postnatal period.

Relevant reflexology treatment

The muscusloskeletal system remains vulnerable for up to 1 year following childbirth; therefore, strong manipulative techniques are not appropriate in a routine postnatal RZT treatment, unless the mother complains of specific discomforts. However, gentle work along the entire reflex zone for the spine, head, neck, shoulders, pelvis, sacroiliac joints, symphysis pubis and knees to tone the musculoskeletal system can be incorporated into the relaxation treatment. Gentle ankle circling will aid pelvic mechanics and a gentle spinal twist, both in the thoracic reflex zone and the lumbosacral zones will release stiffness and help movement. The advanced technique (see Appendix 2) can be useful for releasing tension, easing neck pain and the discomfort from heavy breasts but special attention should be paid to ensuring that the joint at the base of the big toe is thoroughly supported.

Sedation of the coccygeal and sacral reflex zones may suppress pain caused by extension of the coccyx in labour, especially if there has been mild cephalopelvic disproportion (CPD). However, if there is a known coccygeal fracture which has resulted from the CPD, manipulative techniques should be avoided, and care should be taken when working over the reflex zones for the lower spine as there may be acute pain in the local area. Symptoms which developed during pregnancy and which do not spontaneously resolve, for example carpal tunnel syndrome, should also be treated with sedating techniques as appropriate, but if the problem has not resolved within 6 weeks of delivery, medical referral may be necessary (see also Chapter 4).

Special attention should be given to the reflex zones for the shoulder girdle, particularly if the mother has developed the habit of leaning forwards whilst feeding her baby. Obviously, suitable advice about posture and comfort, as well as specific help to facilitate breast feeding, should be given by the midwife as normal, but RZT can also be used to assist in this process. The scapulae, anterior surface of the shoulders, arms and hands, as well as the upper cervical and thoracic vertebrae should all be worked; specific stimulation over the scapulae is acceptable in almost all mothers and will help to eliminate toxins accumulated in this area.

Working over the dorsum of the foot, using bimanual firm, stimulating, sweeping movements from the distal edges to the midline of each foot may help to tone the abdominal musculature, thereby ultimately strengthening the back (this can also be a useful technique during pregnancy if the mother presents with divarification of the rectus sheath).

If the mother has had epidural analgesia in labour, *very gentle* palpation along the spine reflex zones will elicit those points requiring specific sedation; these zones are usually extremely tender, especially those relating to the point of insertion of the epidural cannula, which is usually at the level of the middle lumbar vertebrae. Inadvertently firm pressure can cause a sharp, shooting pain to surge through the foot and leg. If the precise reflex zones are too tender, a more diverse sedation can be applied by resting the palms of the hands over the entire spine zone on each foot. If the mother experiences ongoing back and neck pain this should be treated initially with sedation of the reflex zones but later, more manipulative techniques can be employed, with caution, to realign the entire musculoskeletal system.

When the mother has had her legs in the lithotomy position, for instrumental delivery or the suturing of an episiotomy, it is important to work on the reflex zones for the whole of the pelvis, notably the symphysis pubis (essential if there has been symphysis pubis discomfort in pregnancy), sacroiliac joint and lower spine reflex zones. Sedating techniques will ease pain and discomfort and assist in reducing any inflammation. The reflex zones for the knees may also require sedation if they have been uncomfortable during pregnancy, especially if the mother has gained a large amount of weight.

UTERUS AND RETAINED PRODUCTS OF CONCEPTION

Structural physiology and aetiology

Once the placenta has been delivered at the end of labour, the mother continues to have a substantial vaginal discharge, the *lochia*, which normally lasts for between 10 and 14 days. The lochial discharges constitute the expulsion from the uterus of the remnants of the products of conception, and allow for involution to occur, in which the uterus returns to its non-pregnant shape and position (although not quite its *pre*-pregnant size) by a process of autolysis and ischaemia. This process of self-digestion and reduction in blood supply dissolves the tissues developed during pregnancy into fluid, which must then be excreted via the kidneys (see below, renal system). The usual pattern of blood loss is initially red, sometimes with small blood clots; it gradually changes from red to brown to pink by about 10 to 14 days, and then to a whitish-yellowish discharge, which may persist for several weeks.

Mild contractions of the uterus occur following delivery in an attempt to expedite the expulsion of the remaining products of conception, and are particularly noticeable during breast feeding, as the oxytocic effects on the myoepithelial cells in the breast also impact on the smooth muscle of the uterine myometrium (see breastfeeding, below). For most women these are uncomfortable, but not excessive, although some mothers experience severe "after pains" for some time, particularly those in whom the myometrium has been over-stretched, such as mothers who have already had several babies, or those whose baby weighed more than 4 kg. It is the responsibility of the midwife to examine the placenta and membranes after the delivery to check if it appears complete, as occasionally some tissue can be retained in the uterus. This causes excessive "after pains" as the uterus attempts to expel the retained products, and increases the risks of infection and/or haemorrhage, which can be life-threatening if not adequately and promptly treated with conventional medical methods.

During late pregnancy the uterus has been displaced from being a pelvic to an abdominal organ, and from being central to tilting to the right side, away from the stomach. In the postnatal period the uterus must shrink in size and return to a position of being anteverted and anteflexed, but this is reliant on adequate tone in the supporting muscles and ligaments of the uterus, fallopian tubes and ovaries, which is also related to proper alignment and adequate functioning of the spine and pelvic bones. For example, sacroiliac joint displacement can put tension on the ovarian (round) ligaments, which indirectly affects the support of the uterus; normal repositioning of the uterus is thus influenced by the dynamics of the round ligaments in relation to the sacroiliac joints.

Relevant reflexology treatment

It is not appropriate to use any stimulating movements over the reflex zones for the uterus in the early days after delivery, as this could potentially precipitate haemorrhage, especially if there are any retained products of conception. However, firm sedating work over the lower edges of the heels will help to tone the uterus and pelvic floor. If this is too uncomfortable for the mother in the first few days following delivery, firm holding of the heels, with the palms over the reflex zones for the uterus, will provide a more generalised and diluted pressure.

After an instrumental delivery or a Caesarean section, when pelvic and abdominal pain can understandably be quite severe, gentle calming treatment should be given, which may ease some of the discomfort through the relaxation factor. It is helpful to stimulate the gastrointestinal tract zones gently in a clockwise direction as this may facilitate peristalsis and avoid the paralytic ileus, which can occur after some abdominal surgery. When the mother reports tenderness on specific reflex points, light sedation can be given; however, extreme care should be taken when working over the reflex zones for the uterus and the abdominal musculature as this will be very tender, sometimes to the point of excrutiating pain the first few days. In some cases it may be possible to observe a thin "angry" red line on either the uterus or abdominal reflex zones, which appears to correspond to the incision/suture line. This can be gently sedated, but only to the level of the mother's tolerance.

If the mother experiences "after pains" that do not seem to indicate the presence of retained products, a general relaxation treatment can be given, perhaps while she is feeding the baby. Sometimes, in women who have had several babies, "after pains" can be almost as painful as labour contractions, and RZT can be useful in relieving some of this pain. Treatment can include plenty of "solar plexus" sedation, diaphragm sweeping and general holding. Sedating techniques can be used on the reflex zones for the uterus, ovaries and fallopian tubes, and treatment can be performed for 15 to 20 minutes, several times a day, as necessary (and as time permits). The partner could be shown the basic relaxation techniques so that he can perform short RZT treatments when the mother needs them. On no account should the pituitary gland reflex zones be sedated as this may inhibit breast feeding and interefere with general postnatal physiology.

However, if the uterine fundus is high, there have been excessively large blood clots in the lochia, or there are known retained products still in situ, stimulating movements on the pituitary gland reflex zone can be performed. In these cases, the reflex zone for the uterus will be very tender and may feel quite large, full and bulky in the same way as the midwife's abdominal examination of the mother will reveal a bulky cavity and high fundus. The reflex zones for the urinary tract should also be stimulated to encourage fluid excretion and to allow for extra space for the uterus to normalise its position. The zones for the musculoskeletal system should be manipulated in order to tone the whole area, including the relevant ligaments, to reduce any tensions which may be preventing the uterus from emptying completely and to realign any skeletal displacements. It may also be appropriate to stimulate the Bladder 60 acupressure point to encourage expulsion of the retained products (see Figs 6.1 and 5.2).

PELVIC FLOOR

Structural physiology and aetiology

The vagina, vulva and perineum may have been traumatised during the birth, either from lacerations or an episiotomy; occasionally a severe tear may extend into the anal sphincter, causing more extreme pain and difficulty with defaecation

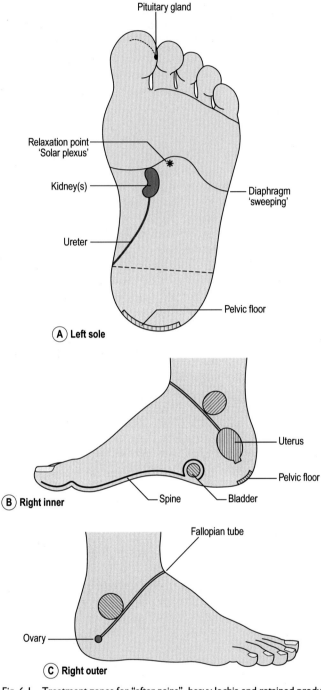

Pituitary gland

Relaxation point
'Solar plexus'

Kidney(s)

Ureter

Diaphragm
'sweeping'

Pelvic floor

(A) Left sole

Uterus

Pelvic floor

(B) Right inner

Spine

Bladder

Fallopian tube

Ovary

(C) Right outer

Fig. 6.1   Treatment zones for "after pains", heavy lochia and retained products;
(A) left sole, (B) right inner, (C) right outer

(see below). Bearing in mind the impact of the musculoskeletal system and the
supporting ligaments on the internal organs, as previously discussed, any
misalignment in the sacrum or hips will influence the function of the cervix
and vagina, whereas the upper segment of the uterus may be affected by displacement of the symphysis pubis and the groin.

The perineum is directly affected by stability of the pelvic joints, especially of the sacroiliac joints, because injury or displacement in this area impacts on the lumbar vertebrae, alters the functioning of the diaphragm and decreases tone in the pelvic floor musculature. Women with poor pelvic floor control are likely to have problems with the mechanics of the bony pelvis; conversely, repetitive dysfunction in the sacroiliac joints, or in those at the lumbosacral or iliolumbar junctions, may be perpetuated or exacerbated by weakness of the pelvic floor. Additionally, damage in one or both sacroiliac joints may adversely affect pelvic floor tone, which then causes diminished movements in the ilium and the ischial tuberosities, leading to further strain on the sacroiliac joints.

Relevant reflexology treatment

Sedation of the specific reflex zones for the perineum, together with drainage of the reflex zones for the lymphatics of the pelvis, can assist in reducing the intensity of pain in a suture line from lacerations or an episiotomy. Any disordered reflex zones, as identified by the mother reporting tenderness at specific points, or by the practitioner becoming aware of irregularities in the pelvic zones, should be treated with mild sedation. This includes the pelvic floor (perineum), pelvic supports and organs, together with the abdominal musculature. Sedation of any spinal reflex zones which appear disordered should be undertaken, and the advanced technique (see Appendix 2) should be applied gently, without any excessive manipulative movements, to the length of the spinal column, to realign the musculoskeletal system. Whilst these techniques will not directly aid wound healing, their intention is to restore homeostasis, which will indirectly facilitate all aspects of recovery. It is also wise to work right out to the posterior edge of each heel to include the reflex zones for the anal sphincter with sedating techniques to ease tenderness resulting from bruising, stretching and any haemorrhoids which may be present (see also Chapter 4) (see Fig. 6.2).

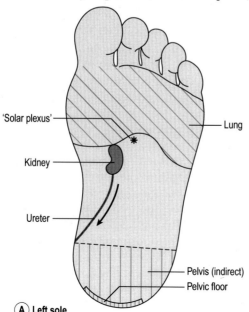

Fig. 6.2 Treatment zones for pelvic floor and urinary problems;
(A) left sole (B) right inner

Continued

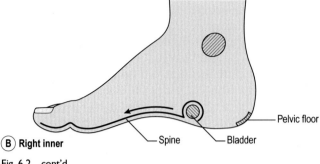

(B) **Right inner**

Fig. 6.2   cont'd

KIDNEYS, BLADDER AND MICTURITION

Structural physiology and aetiology

The kidneys are particularly active in the first days of the puerperium as there is an increase in the quantity of urine being excreted, due to the excess fluid from the autolysis, which is a part of the process of involution of the uterus (see above). Often, the amount of urine to be excreted is too much for the kidneys to cope with immediately, and the excess fluid escapes into the extracellular tissues, exacerbating any oedema already present. As the kidneys gradually excrete the fluid over the next few days, the oedema, especially in the ankles, will diminish and the legs will return to their normal size.

Structurally, the bladder is supported by the medial umbilical ligaments and the urachus – the vestigial remnant of the umbilical cord. The urachus is fused to the inner linea alba, but is flexible to allow mobility of the bladder; this is often disrupted during incision for Caesarean section, predisposing women to bladder prolapse or irritation of the superior bladder wall. The mechanics of the bladder neck are influenced by the pubocervical ligaments and movement or extension of the vagina, as in childbirth. The lowest part of the urethra and the urethral sphincter is embedded in the urogenital diaphragm and is supported by the pubovesical and pubourethral ligaments; the urethra is also linked to vaginal movement, length and tone.

There is a reflex relationship between the bladder and the lower ribs and lumbosacral spine, between the kidneys and the thoracolumbar junction, and between the urethra and the lumbosacral and coccygeal spine. Furthermore, there is a direct relationship between the kidneys and the psoas muscle, which is "one of the most marked within whole body mechanics" (Stone 2007:159), so tension in the kidneys can affect distal parts of the body including the base of the skull, the sacroiliac joints, hips and lower limbs. Similarly, there is a close relationship between the renal system and the respiratory system, the kidneys and lungs being separated geographically only by the diaphragm, and both organs being developed from the same germ layer. The surrounding bony structures, i.e. the ribcage, thoracic and lumbar spine regions will also impact on the position and wellbeing of the relevant internal organs. Stone (2000:159) notes also that many cervicobrachial restrictions are interlinked with renal dysfunction, as the renal fascia is supplied by the phrenic nerve;

kidney irritation may, therefore, present as mid-cervical spine irritation, with referred pain at the level of the third to the fifth cervical vertebrae, which affects skin and the musculature of the neck and upper shoulder girdle.

Bladder function is commonly disrupted after the birth, not least because the mother experiences pain and discomfort, which interfere with her normal excretory activity. The progress of the mother's labour, or the delivery process, occasionally results in trauma to the bladder or urethra, particularly when there has been a prolonged labour with the fetus in an abnormal position, or an instrumental delivery such as the use of forceps, a ventouse extraction, breech birth or twin delivery. During micturition the pelvic floor relaxes, the bladder descends and the bladder neck moves away from the internal surface of the symphysis pubis; after micturition the pelvic floor contracts and the organs revert to their normal positions. However, scars, suture lines and pelvic floor weakness following childbirth, and displacement of the symphysis pubis, as in gestational diastasis, interfere with this reflex mechanism and may lead to incontinence, urgency or frequency of micturition (in the absence of any infection). Pelvic floor weakness prevents the muscles from relaxing and contracting appropriately, which may cause a neurogenic obstruction in the bladder neck or urethra, making it more difficult to pass urine, and leading to retention of urine. The detrusor muscle of the bladder becomes overstretched or may have been damaged during instrumental or operative delivery, especially when neighbouring ligaments and connective tissues have also been traumatised, and this can lead to retention with urinary overflow.

Incontinence is particularly common in mothers who have required catheterisation of the bladder either during normal labour or prior to Caesarean section, but even after normal delivery, the mother may experience bladder spasm due to irritation of the lining when the bladder is overfull. At a local level, the straining required to empty an over-distended bladder will eventually lead to hypertrophy and irritation of the bladder wall and, ultimately, to incontinence, which may become a chronic condition, which in some women lasts into the menopause; the long-term sequelae of childbearing on the urinary system are often disregarded because women are embarrassed to discuss them. Regionally, any nerve damage in the spinal cord at the level of the bladder will also affect bladder function, so women who have had a spinal anaesthetic for a Caesarean section are particularly at risk. Osteopaths believe that somatic structures which send nerve fibres to the second to third sacral segment of the spine influence the neural reflex arc, and that any disruption to these structures may, therefore, present as problems in the feet, which are linked to the first and second sacral vertebrae. In relation to osteopathic treatment, Stone (2005:267) comments that: *"even if the patient's foot is the only part treated, there may be an effect on the bladder, strange as it may seem!"* – although this is, of course, of no surprise to reflexologists!

Women also continue to be prone to urinary tract infection in the puerperium, although for slightly differing reasons than those in pregnancy. Muscles and organs have been stretched during pregnancy and further traumatised during birth. Inflammation and bruising leads to the area being prone to invasion by bacteria, plus contamination of the urethral meatus from the lochia increases the risk of ascending infection. A tendency to cystitis or recurrent bladder infection may also be due to pelvic congestion, causing irritability and contraction of the bladder, leading to incomplete emptying and retention of urine, inflammation of local tissues and an increased incidence of infection.

Relevant reflexology treatment

Reflexology has been shown to increase renal circulation (Sudmeier et al 1999) and a systematic review found it to be effective in alleviating urinary symptoms in people with multiple sclerosis (Wang et al 2008). A randomised controlled trial by Mak et al (2007) demonstrated a reduction in the daytime frequency of micturition in women who had over-activity of the detrusor muscle, compared to women who received basic foot massage, although the overall 24-hour frequency was not statistically significant. Anecdotal evidence appears to suggest that reflexology does have an effect on the urinary system, although whether this is mechanical, neurological, chemical or psychological is difficult to determine.

In the early puerperium the commonest problem is retention of urine, with or without overflow. In addition to a generalised relaxation treatment, stimulation of the reflex zones for the whole renal tract should be performed, but it is *essential* to work *from* the kidney reflex zone *to* the ureter and on to the bladder zone to avoid ascending infection. On no account should "caterpillar walking" or stimulating movements be performed in the opposite direction from bladder to kidney reflex zone. Stimulation of any of these reflex zones may, however, be painful for the mother, especially the kidney reflex zones, and it is preferable to perform very short treatments of 3 to 5 minutes repeated every 20 to 30 minutes than to attempt to complete a full treatment if the mother is unable to tolerate it. Techniques to encourage decongestion of the pelvic circulation and lymphatics include ankle circling, brisk bimanual effleurage of the heels and vigorous massage across the reflex zone for the pelvic lymphatics on the feet; the mother can be advised to perform "wrist wringing" movements every half an hour or so.

Manipulative manoeuvres and the advanced technique (see Appendix 2) will help to realign the musculoskeletal system and ease any tensions and torsions which may be complicating the situation. These should include the whole of the spine, but in this case the "caterpillar crawling" should start from the reflex zones for the coccygeal end of the spine, working up through the sacral, lumbar and thoracic to the cervical vertebrae to encourage homeostatic balance between the sacrum and the cranium. The whole of the pelvis should be worked, with sedation of any painful reflex zones, especially the sacroiliac joints and symphysis pubis, plus the reflex zones for the ribs and diaphragm, to encompass all the reflex arcs and related areas of the body. Similarly, the links with the respiratory system suggest that toning movements over the reflex zones for the lungs and nasopharynx can be useful and may avoid the mother requiring catheterisation (Marquardt 2000:193) (see Fig. 6.3).

For longer-term treatment of incontinence, most probably by reflexologists in independent practice, specific attention should be given to the reflex zones for the renal tract (kidneys, ureters, bladder), anal sphincter, pelvic floor and abdominal musculature, sacroiliac joint, symphysis pubis and the entire spine. Initial sessions should be given fairly lightly to stimulate the organs, then

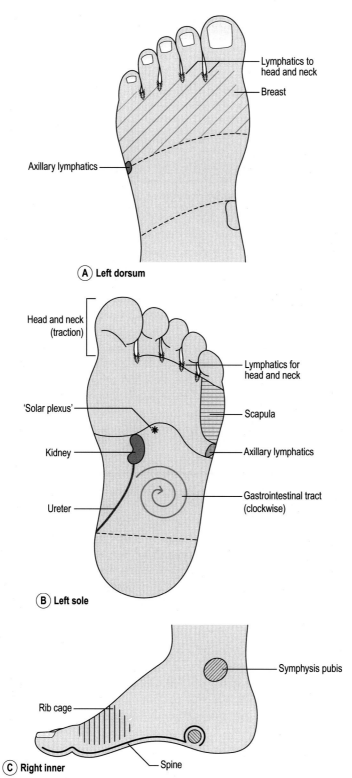

Fig. 6.3   Treatment zones for lactation problems; (A) left dorsum, (B) left sole, (C) right inner

increased pressure should be applied as the course of treatments continues, to tone the area. Marquardt (2000:193) refers to this as the Arndt-Schultz rule, in which "weak impulses stimulate, strong ones retard, very strong ones paralyse".

NB These treatments can also be applied, with caution, during pregnancy, if the mother suffers from acute urinary retention due to incarceration of a retroverted gravid uterus.

GASTROINTESTINAL TRACT AND DEFAECATION

Structural physiology and aetiology

Constipation is a physical and psycho-emotional problem of the puerperium, not least because the mother may feel frightened of pain on defaecation due to perineal and anal damage, as well as possibly being inhibited whilst an in-patient in the postnatal ward at the hospital. In addition she will probably not have eaten a great deal in the last few days leading up to delivery, as many women experience a reduction in appetite, and often report loose bowel movements immediately before the onset of labour. Furthermore, if she suffered haemorrhoids during pregnancy, or if the mode of delivery exacerbated any to the point of prolapse, anal sphincter trauma will also inhibit pelvic floor function, leading to retention of rectal contents. If the mother has had a Caesarean section she may experience paralytic ileus, in which internal abdominal trauma temporarily impairs peristalsis within the gut, preventing the passage of food towards the rectum.

Constipation may be related to uncoordinated reflexes in the gastrointestinal tract and/or to pelvic floor muscle weakness. Anatomically, the stomach is supported by ligaments which are essentially one extended structure. The greater omentum connects the stomach to the diaphragm, spleen, kidney and gall bladder, and the lesser omentum connects the oesophagus, bile duct, portal vein and numerous nerves and lymphatics, which allow the stomach to swing freely under the diaphragm and liver. The duodenum is linked to the posterior abdominal wall by the renal fascia, psoas muscle and the arcuate ligament to the right of the diaphragm, then indirectly to the upper lumbar spine on the right, while the rest of the small intestine, the jejunum and ileum are attached indirectly to the anterior surface of the third lumbar vertebra. The large intestine is attached to the renal fascia, psoas muscle, diaphragm and cystoduodenal ligament; the rectum is attached posteriorly to the sacrum and the anal sphincter is attached via the anococcygeal raphe to the coccyx posteriorly and the perineal body anteriorly. Numerous other ligamentous structures also help to support the gastrointestinal tract so that it maintains its position, flexibility and mobility. There are neural links too, between the vagus nerve and thoracic nerves, impacting on the lumbar, thoracic and cervical vertebrae, the ribs and, for the rectum and anus, the lumbar, sacral and coccygeal vertebrae. Thus, the gastrointestinal tract is influenced by whole-body mechanics.

Constipation is often accompanied by headaches, which may be argued in conventional terms to be due to the accumulated toxins and waste, but which may also be related to the mechanical links between the gut and the head and neck including the vagus nerve, cervical vertebrae and mesenteric artery.

Alternatively, or sometimes in addition, poor gut motility is accompanied by backache, especially during pregnancy and after delivery. These symptoms should not be seen in isolation but should be considered as part of the whole structural aetiology; while the individual symptoms may be treated separately, they constitute part of the whole-person management.

Relevant reflexology treatment

At a basic level, peristalsis can be encouraged with clockwise massage of the arches of the feet or the palms of the hands, in the areas related to the reflex zones for the intestines. This can easily be taught to mothers for self-administration and it is also a useful treatment for colic in the neonate. Massage should always be in a clockwise direction to accommodate the direction of peristalsis. If treatment is given by the midwife or reflexologist, the reflex zones for the abdominal musculature and the entire internal abdominal organs can be stimulated, including the rectum and anus. However, if the mother has concomitant haemorrhoids, sedation of the reflex zone for the anal sphincter should be performed to ease pain. The fist can be placed under the diaphragm line so that the knuckles rest securely under this area, then very firm pressure with the knuckles stationary while the wrist moves clockwise can be comforting and effective in providing further stimulation to the gastrointestinal tract.

Manipulation of the reflex zones for the musculoskeletal system should include the advanced technique (see Appendix 2), then "caterpillar walking" down the entire spine zone, sedating any specific painful areas as they are found. Manipulation of the spine and ribs, and sedation of the sacroiliac joint and symphysis pubis may also be necessary; in addition, ankle circling, to encourage mobility in the hips, will also tone the attachments.

LACTATION AND BREASTFEEDING

Structural physiology and aetiology

It is essential to understand the physiology of lactation in order to adminster RZT correctly. Many reflexologists incorrectly assume that lactation can be stimulated by working over the breast reflex zones, but this is not entirely true as the hormones for lactation originate from the pituitary gland. Expulsion of the placenta in the third stage of labour removes from the mother's body the hormones which were present in large amounts during pregnancy, notably oestrogen and progesterone. As the oestrogen levels subside, prolactin levels in the anterior pituitary gland increase and trigger the acini cells in the breast to produce milk from the fatty globules in the mother's blood. When the baby is put to suckle at the breast a "let down" reflex occurs in which the posterior pituitary gland releases oxytocin which causes contraction of the muscular myoepithelial cells surrounding the acini cells. This causes the milk cells to be squeezed so that milk is pushed along the ducts towards the nipple. As the baby removes milk from the breasts, further prolactin is produced to supply more milk, and the "let down" mechanism triggers further release of oxytocin. Thus this cycle of events continues and a supply and demand situation is established.

However, whilst it is not usually necessary to stimulate directly the reflex zones for the breasts in order to facilitate lactation, there is a theory that insertion of an intravenous cannula into the back of the hand can suppress the breast reflex zone on that hand, possibly causing difficulties in establishing lactation on the affected side. This has not been proven with any formal research but anecdotally has been seen to hold true and it would be interesting to investigate further. In the early days of the puerperium there is little colostrum in the breasts, the milk coming into the breasts on about the third or fourth day, often causing engorgement and resulting tenderness and discomfort. If this tenderness becomes excessive in one isolated segment of the breast tissue it may indicate an abscess in one lobe; this may also be observed on the dorsum of the relevant foot, in one section of the breast reflex zone, which appears red and "angry" and feels hot to the touch.

Structurally, any factors that impact on the anterior or posterior chest wall, the thoracic cavity, shoulder girdle or head and neck, may adversely affect the breasts, or vice versa. This has already been seen in relation to pregnancy (see Chapter 4). Furthermore, the intimate relationship between the upper and lower spine means that pelvic alterations in labour may impact on the thoracic vertebrae, influencing the breasts, and tension on the neck will put strain on the brain and, indirectly, on the pituitary gland. It is known that many new mothers experience upper back and neck ache during the early days of breast feeding, simply from incorrect posture, i.e. bending forwards so that the breast reaches the baby, rather than lifting the baby up to put him to the breast. This pain will be accentuated if the breasts are particularly large and heavy, or if there is any history of neck and upper spinal misalignment.

Relevant reflexology treatment

During general relaxation treatments the breast reflex zones do not, physiologically, need to be stimulated directly, and can be uncomfortable, especially in the early days. However, if the mother has lactation difficulties, she can be advised to massage over the corresponding area of the hands, between the tendons below the fingers on the dorsal surface of the hands, to tone the breast area. This can be performed every 3–4 hours, or whenever she remembers to do it. The breast reflex zones on the feet can also be worked with the "caterpillar crawling" movements. If lactation is slow or poor, despite correct and adequate positioning of the baby at the breast, stimulation of the pituitary gland will encourage production of oxytocin to facilitate the cycle of production and "let down".

Manipulative movements of the upper spine, head, neck, shoulders and central thoracic spine zones, with specific stimulation to the reflex zones for the cervical vertebrae, assist in loosening the musculoskeletal system and aiding neurological interconnections. The reflex zones for the lungs can also be stimulated to aid homeostasis in the chest area in general and the treatment should include repeated diaphragm sweeping. Drainage and stimulation of the lymphatics for the head and neck and the axillae will also aid homeostasis. In truth, general relaxation treatments are sometimes sufficient, especially when mothers are stressed about breast feeding, because the cortisol–oxytocin relationship is rebalanced. Some midwives have effectively employed simple relaxation techniques during breast feeding in mothers whose babies are in the special care baby unit (personal communications with midwives), and Tipping (2000:147–157) advocates this practice to reduce stress, fear and anxiety.

CASE STUDY 6.1   POOR "LET DOWN" REFLEX

Jayne was a 39-year-old obese lady whose first baby had been delivered by Caesarean section at 35 weeks of pregnancy due to fulminating pre-eclampsia. Although he was healthy for his gestational age and was breathing unaided, he was admitted to the special care baby unit for observation. Jayne recovered quickly from the immediate effects of the operation, but her blood pressure remained labile and mobility was slow. She was also very upset at the chain of events and felt that she had "failed" her baby by not having a normal birth. She was, therefore, desperate to breastfeed him, but fixing him to the breast was complicated by the large size of her breasts and a slightly immature sucking reflex. This added to her sense of failure and adversely affected her manual dexterity when positioning her baby at the breast, all of which contributed to a poor "let down" reflex and an inadequate milk supply and, after having initially lost weight, the baby had not yet started to regain his birth weight.

On the sixth day after the birth, reflex zone therapy (RZT) was offered by the lactation specialist midwife, who performed a general relaxation treatment whilst Jayne had her baby fixed on the breast. Specific attention was paid to the endocrine and renal systems, the lymphatics and the gastrointestinal tract (Jayne was suffering from constipation and flatus). After only 10 minutes Jayne noticeably relaxed and starting talking quietly to her baby, something she had not done on previous days. It was also observed that she spontaneously adjusted her own and the baby's position so that she was holding him more securely. The baby had been suckling but appearing not to obtain much milk, but after a further few minutes he started to suck voraciously, a fact which caused Jayne to start crying. Treatments were continued for the next few feeds and Jayne's milk supply increased exponentially; within 2 more days the baby had put on more weight. The success of the RZT was attributed to a reduction in anxiety and an increase in Jayne's self-confidence, which positively affected her "let down" reflex, increased oxytocin production and facilitated an improvement in the milk supply.

In the event of excessive milk supply, especially in the first few days after delivery, the breast zones can be very briefly sedated, but it is not appropriate to sedate the pituitary gland zones as the intention is to regulate, rather than suppress, milk production. However, an overall relaxation treatment in which the endocrine gland zones are treated, and the axillary lymphatics are drained can facilitate this regulation without adversely disturbing the physiology of lactation. It is also useful to stimulate the reflex zones for the urinary tract to

Structural reflex zone therapy for the puerperium

aid kidney function, and for the intestinal zones to facilitate excretion via the bowels. Milk engorgement can be treated with these techniques plus stimulation of the reflex zones for the lower cervical and upper thoracic vertebrae (C7 to T7), and sedation of the "solar plexus" and sternum; a diversified suppression of the entire breast reflex area with the hands on both feet may also help.

If the mother is experiencing any tenderness at the nipple, the reflex zone in the centre of the breast zone will be acutely tender to touch and can be sedated. Sore nipples cannot be treated directly with RZT, although this sedation may reduce pain and tenderness, and the rebalancing and relaxing effects may indirectly aid homeostasis. Since the suspensory ligament of the nipple runs across the fifth rib and links to the pectoral muscle and sternum, manipulation of the reflex zones for the neck, shoulder girdle, ribcage, diaphragm and axillary lymphatics will help to improve circulation and drainage within the breasts, release tension in the connective tissues and ducts and ease any nerve irritation which may accompany the problem.

If a breast abscess develops or mastitis occurs, it is not professionally appropriate to use RZT to treat this condition; the practitioner should refer to the midwife who should employ normal midwifery management, with or without medical prescription of antibiotics as necessary. Once the initial symptoms have subsided RZT can be given for relaxation and to ease pain, but should not focus on either stimulating or sedating the specific reflex zones.

If the mother is considering ceasing breast feeding *no* stimulation of the breast or pituitary gland reflex zones should be undertaken, as this would increase the oxytocin and continue, or even complicate, the process of suppression. The general relaxation treatment can be given, with lymphatic drainage as before, and stimulation of the renal and gastrointestinal tracts. Plenty of relaxing holds and techniques such as diaphragm sweeping and "solar plexus" sedation should be used throughout the treatment; gentle work over the heart and lung zones may also calm the mother and help her emotionally come to terms with her decision to feed her baby artificially.

References

Agren A, Berg M: Tactile massage and severe nausea and vomiting during pregnancy – women's experiences, *Scand J Caring Sci* 20(2):169–176, 2006.

Asamura N, Nozomu Y, Hiroyuki S: 1998 Selectively stimulating skin receptors for tactile display Virtual Reality 32.7; cited in Tiran D Chummun H 2005 The physiological basis of reflexology and its use as a diagnostic tool, *Complement Ther Clin Pract* 11(1):58–64, 1998.

Ascari L, Corradi P, Beccai L, et al: A miniaturized and flexible optoelectronic sensing system for tactile skin, *J Micromech Microeng* 17:2288–2298, 2007.

Baerheim A, Algrøy R, Skogedal KR, et al: Feet – a diagnostic tool? *Tidsskr Nor Laegeforen* 118(5):753–755, 1998.

Baldry P: *Acupuncture trigger points and musculoskeletal pain*, ed 3, Edinburgh, 2005, Churchill Livingstone.

Bamigboye AA, Smyth R: Interventions for varicose veins and leg oedema in pregnancy, *Cochrane Database Syst Rev* 24(1): CD001066, 2007.

Bastard J, Tiran D: Aromatherapy and massage for antenatal anxiety: its effect on the fetus, *Complement Ther Clin Pract* 12(1):48–54, 2006.

Bello D, White–Traut R, Schwertz D, et al: An exploratory study of neurohormonal responses of healthy men to massage, *J Altern Complement Med* 14(4):387–394, 2008.

Bender T, Nagy G, Barna I, et al: The effect of physical therapy on beta-endorphin levels, *Eur J Appl Physiol* 100(4):371–382, 2007.

Berglund A, Alfredsson L, Jensen I, et al: The association between exposure to a rear-end collision and future health complaints, *J Clin Epidemiol* 54(8):851–856, 2001.

Birch S: Trigger point – acupuncture point correlations revisited, *J Altern Complement Med* 9(1):91–103, 2003.

Billhult A, Lindholm C, Gunnarsson R, et al: The effect of massage on cellular immunity, endocrine and psychological factors in women with breast cancer – A randomized controlled clinical trial, *Auton Neurosci* 140(1–2):88–95, 2008.

Bishop E, McKinnon E, Weir E, et al: Reflexology in the management of encopresis and chronic constipation, *Paediatr Nurs* 15(3):20–21, 2003.

Booth L: Vertical reflexology, *Positive Health* 63 (April), 2001. Available online at www.positivehealth.com/article–view.php?articleid=1383. Accessed March 3, 2009.

Booth L: Vertical reflex therapy (VRT) for sports injuries, *Positive Health* 134 (April), 2007. Available online at www.positivehealth.com/article–abstract.php?articleid=2084. Accessed 3 March 2009.

Brown CA, Lido C: Reflexology treatment for patients with lower limb amputations and phantom limb pain – an exploratory pilot study, *Complement Ther Clin Pract* 14(2):124–131, 2008.

Bull L: Sunflower therapy for children with specific learning difficulties (dyslexia): a randomised, controlled trial, *Complement Ther Clin Pract* 13(1):15–24, 2007.

Chang SB, Park YW, Cho JS, et al: Differences of cesarean section rates according to San–Yin–Jiao(SP6) acupressure for women in labor, *Taehan Kanho Hakhoe Chi* 34(2):324–332, 2004.

Chang MY, Wang SY, Chen CH: Effects of massage on pain and anxiety during labour: a randomized controlled trial in Taiwan, *J Adv Nurs* 38(1):68–73, 2002.

Chen LL, Su YC, Su CH, et al: Acupressure and meridian massage: combined effects on increasing body weight in premature infants, *J Clin Nurs* 17(9):1174–1181, 2008.

Chinappi AS Jr, Getzoff H: Chiropractic/dental cotreatment of lumbosacral pain with temporomandibular joint involvement, *J Manipulative Physiol Ther* 19(9):607–612, 1996.

Choi GS, Han JB, Park JH, et al: Effects of moxibustion to zusanli (ST36) on alteration of natural killer cell activity in rats, *Am J Chin Med* 32(2):303–312, 2004.

Collinge W, Kahn J, Yarnold P, et al: Couples and cancer: feasibility of brief instruction in massage and touch therapy to build caregiver efficacy, *J Soc Integr Oncol* 5(4):147–154, 2007.

Coulson C, Jenkins J: Complementary and alternative medicine utilisation in NHS and private clinic settings: a United Kingdom survey of 400 infertility patients, *J Exp Clin Assist Reprod* 2(1):5, 2005.

Crane B: *Reflexology: the definitive practitioner's manual*, London, 1997, Element.

Cwikel J, Gidron Y, Sheiner E: Psychological interactions with infertility among women, *Eur J Obstet Gynecol Reprod Biol* 117(2):126–131, 2004.

Damany S, Bellis J: *It's not carpal tunnel syndrome: RSI theory and therapy for computer professionals*, Philadelphia, 2000, Simax.

Davis CG: Injury threshold: whiplash-associated disorders, *J Manipulative Physiol Ther* 23(6):420–427, 2000.

Diego MA, Jones NA, Field T, et al: Maternal psychological distress, prenatal cortisol, and fetal weight, *Psychosom Med* 68(5):747–753, 2006.

Dougans I: *The new reflexology a unique blend of traditional Chinese medicine and Western reflexology practice for better health and healing*, New York, 2006, Marlowe and Co.

Dung H, Vlogston CP, Dunn JW: *Acupuncture – an anatomical approach*, London, 2004, CRC Press.

Ejindu A: The effects of foot and facial massage on sleep induction, blood pressure, pulse and respiratory rate: crossover pilot study, *Complement Ther Clin Pract* 13(4):266–275, 2007.

Enzer S: *Reflexology, a tool for midwives*, Australia, 2000, Self-published.

Ernst E, Resch KL: Concept of true and perceived placebo effects, *BMJ* 311(7004):551–553, 1995.

Feder E, Liisberg GB, Lenstrup C, et al: Zonal therapy in relation to women in childbirth, *Jordemodern* 107(5):168–170, 1994.

Field T: Pregnancy and labor alternative therapy research, *Altern Ther Health Med* 14(5): 28–34, 2008.

Field T, Diego M, Cullen C, et al: Fibromyalgia pain and substance P decrease and sleep improves after massage therapy, *J Clin Rheumatol* 8(2):72–76, 2002.

Field T, Hernandez-Reif M, Diego M, et al: Cortisol decreases and serotonin and dopamine increase following massage therapy, *Int J Neurosci* 115(10):1397–1413, 2005.

Field T, Hernandez-Reif M, Diego M, et al: Stability of mood states and biochemistry across pregnancy, *Infant Behav Dev* 29(2):262–267, 2006.

Field T, Figueiredo B, Hernandez-Reif M, et al: Massage therapy reduces pain in pregnant women, alleviates prenatal depression in both parents and improves their relationships, *J Bodyw Mov Ther* 12(2):146–150, 2008.

Field T, Diego M, Hernandez-Reif M: Prematurity and potential predictors, *Int J Neurosci* 118(2):277–289, 2008b.

Frey Law LA, Evans S, Knudtson J, et al: Massage reduces pain perception and hyperalgesia in experimental muscle pain: a randomized. Controlled trial, *J Pain* 9(8):714–721, 2008. Epub 2 May 2008.

Friedman MH, Weisberg J: The craniocervical connection: a retrospective analysis of 300 whiplash patients with cervical and temporomandibular disorders, *Cranio* 18(3):163–167, 2000.

Fujita M, Endoh Y, Saimon N, et al: Effect of massaging babies on mothers: pilot study on the changes in mood states and salivary cortisol level, *Complement Ther Clin Pract* 12(3):181–185, 2006.

Garner B, Phillips LJ, Schmidt HM, et al: Pilot study evaluating the effect of massage therapy on stress, anxiety and aggression in a young adult psychiatric inpatient unit, *Aust N Z J Psychiatry* 42(5):414–422, 2008.

Gaudernack LC, Forbord S, Hole E: Acupuncture administered after spontaneous rupture of membranes at term significantly reduces the length of birth and use of oxytocin. A randomized controlled trial, *Acta Obstet Gynecol Scand* 85(11):1348–1353, 2006.

Gaudet LM, Dyzak R, Aung SK, et al: Effectiveness of acupuncture for the initiation of labour at term: a pilot randomized controlled trial, *J Obstet Gynaecol Can* 30(12):1118–23, 2008.

Gustafsson J, Nilsson-Wikmar L: Influence of specific muscle training on pain, activity limitation and kinesiophobia in women with back pain post-partum – a 'single-subject research design', *Physiother Res Int* 13(1):18–30, 2008.

Harper TC, Coeytaux RR, Chen W, et al: A randomized controlled trial of acupuncture for initiation of labor in nulliparous women, *J Matern Fetal Neonatal Med* 19(8):465–470, 2006.

Hernandez-Reif M, Field T, Krasnegor J, et al: Children with cystic fibrosis benefit from massage therapy, *J Pediatr Psychol* 24(2):175–181, 1999.

Hernandez-Reif M, Ironson G, Field T, et al: Breast cancer patients have improved immune and neuroendocrine functions following massage therapy, *J Psychosom Res* 57(1):45–52, 2004.

Hodgson DM, Nakamura T, Walker AK: Prophylactic role for complementary and alternative medicine in perinatal programming of adult health, *Forsch Komplementmed* 14(2):92–101, 2007.

Holt J, Lord J, Acharya U, et al: The effectiveness of foot reflexology in inducing ovulation: a sham-controlled randomized trial, *Fertil Steril* Jun 18, 2008.

House of Lords Select Committee on Science and Technology: *Sixth report on Complementary and Alternative Medicine*, London, 2000, HMSO.

Ingham E, Byers D: *The original works of Eunice Ingham: Stories the feet can tell thru reflexology and stories the feet have told thru reflexology*, ed 2, USA, 1992, Ingham Publishing Inc.

Ingram J, Domagala C, Yates S: The effects of shiatsu on post-term pregnancy, *Complement Ther Med* 13(1):11–5, 2005.

Janovsky B, White AR, Filshie J, et al: Are acupuncture points tender? A blinded study of Spleen 6, *J Altern Complement Med* 6(2):149–155, 2000.

Jewell D, Young G: Interventions for nausea and vomiting in early pregnancy, *Cochrane Database Syst Rev* (4): CD000145, 2003.

Kao MJ, Hsieh YL, Kuo FJ, et al: Electrophysiological assessment of acupuncture points, *Am J Phys Med Rehabil* 85(5):443–448, 2006.

Kellgren JH: Observations on referred pain arising from muscle, *Clin Sci* 3 :175–190, 1938. Cited in Baldry PE: *Acupuncture, trigger points and musculoskeletal pain*, ed 3, Edinburgh, 2005, Elsevier.

Kellgren JH: On the distribution of pain arising from deep somatic structures with charts of segmental pain areas, *Clin Sci* 4 :35–46, 1939. Cited in Baldry PE: *Acupuncture, trigger points and musculoskeletal pain*, ed 3, Edinburgh, 2005, Elsevier.

Kim YS, Kim MZ, Jeong IS: The effect of self-foot reflexology on the relief of premenstrual syndrome and dysmenorrhea in high school girls, *Taehan Kanho Hakhoe Chi* 34(5):801–808, 2004.

Kimber L, McNabb M, Mc Court C, et al: Massage or music for pain relief in labour: a pilot randomised placebo controlled trial, *Eur J Pain* 12(8):961–969, 2008.

Kissinger J, Kaczmarek L: Healing touch and fertility: a case report, *Journal of Perinatal Education* 15(2):13–20, 2006.

Kohara H, Miyauchi T, Suehiro Y, et al: Combined modality treatment of aromatherapy, footsoak, and reflexology relieves fatigue in patients with cancer, *J Palliat Med* 7(6): 791–796, 2004.

Kristjansson E, Jónsson H Jr: Is the sagittal configuration of the cervical spine changed in women with chronic whiplash syndrome? A comparative computer-assisted radiographic assessment, *J Manipulative Physiol Ther* 25(9):550–555, 2002.

Lambert MC: *Finding your feet: an introduction to the metamorphic technique*, London, 1988, Lambert (self published).

Lavelle ED, Lavelle W, Smith HS: Myofascial trigger points, *Anesthesiol Clin* 25(4):841–851, 2007.

Laurence JA, French PW, Lindner RA, et al:Biological effects of electromagnetic fields – mechanisms for the effects of pulsed microwave radiation on protein conformation, *J Theor Biol* 206(2):291–298, 2000.

Lee YM: Effect of self-foot reflexology massage on depression, stress responses and immune functions of middle aged women, *Taehan Kanho Hakhoe Chi* 36(1):179–88, 2006.

Lee MK, Chang SB, Kang DH: Effects of SP6 acupressure on labor pain and length of delivery time in women during labor, *J Altern Complement Med* 10(6):959–965, 2004.

Lett A: *Reflex zone therapy for health professionals*, London, 2000, Churchill Livingstone.

Luo F, Wang JY: Modulation of central nociceptive coding by acupoint stimulation, *Neurochem Res* 33(10): 1950–1955, 2008.

Mackereth PA, Booth K, Hillier VF, et al: Reflexology and progressive muscle relaxation training for people with multiple sclerosis: a crossover trial, *Complement Ther Clin Pract* 15(1):14–21, 2009.

Magill L, Berenson S: The conjoint use of music therapy and reflexology with hospitalized advanced stage cancer patients and their families, *Palliat Support Care* 6(3):289–296, 2008.

Mak HL, Cheon WC, Wong T, et al: Randomized controlled trial of foot reflexology for patients with symptomatic idiopathic detrusor overactivity, *Int Urogynecol J Pelvic Floor Dysfunct* 18(6):653–658, 2007.

Makino Y, Shinoda H: Selective stimulation to skin receptors by suction pressure control SICE, *Annual Conference Proceedings* 3:2103–2108, 2004.

Marquardt H: *Reflex zone therapy of the feet: A textbook for therapists*, Northampton, 1983, Thorsons.

Marquardt H: *Reflexotherapy of the feet*, Stuttgart, 2000, Thieme.

McNabb MT, Kimber L, Haines A, et al: Does regular massage from late pregnancy to birth decrease maternal pain perception during labour and birth? – A feasibility study to investigate a programme of massage, controlled breathing and visualization, from 36 weeks of pregnancy until birth, *Complement Ther Clin Pract* 12(3):222–231, 2006.

McNeill JA, Alderdice FA, McMurray F: A retrospective cohort study exploring the relationship between antenatal reflexology and intranatal outcomes, *Complement Ther Clin Pract* 12(2):119–125, 2006.

McVicar AJ, Greenwood CR, Fewell F, et al: Evaluation of anxiety, salivary cortisol and melatonin secretion following reflexology treatment: a pilot study in healthy individuals, *Complement Ther Clin Pract* 13(3):137–145, 2007.

Medela 2006 – see www.medelabreastfeedingus.com/for-professionals/cbe–information/106/breast–anatomy–research. Breast anatomy research. Accessed January 2, 2009.

Meissner K, Distel H, Mitzdorf U: Evidence for placebo effects on physical but not on biochemical outcome parameters: a review of clinical trials, *BMC Med* 19(5):3, 2007.

Melzack R, Wall PD: Pain mechanisms: a new theory, *Science* 150:971–979, 1965.

Middleditch A, Oliver J: *Functional anatomy of the spine*, ed 2, Edinburgh, 2005, Elsevier.

Minagawa M, Narita J, Tada T, et al: Mechanisms underlying immunologic states during pregnancy: possible association of the sympathetic nervous system, *Cell Immunol* 196(1):1–13, 1999.

Mitchinson AR, Kim HM, Rosenberg JM, et al: Acute postoperative pain management using massage as an adjuvant therapy: a randomized trial, *Arch Surg* 142(12): 1158–1167, 2007.

Mollart L: Single-blind trial addressing the differential effects of two reflexology techniques versus rest, on ankle and foot oedema in late pregnancy, *Complement Ther Nurs Midwifery* 9(4):203–208, 2003.

Moraska A, Chandler C: Changes in clinical parameters in patients with tension-type headache following massage therapy: a pilot study, *J Man Manip Ther* 16(2): 106–112, 2008.

Motha G, McGrath J: The effects of reflexology on labour outcome, *Journal of Association of Reflexologists* 2:4, 1993.

Mur E, Schmidseder J, Egger I, et al: Influence of reflex zone therapy of the feet on intestinal blood flow measured by color Doppler sonography, *Forsch Komplementarmed Klass Naturheilkd* 8(2):86–89, 2001.

Nakamaru T, Miura N, Fukushima A, et al: Somatotopical relationships between cortical activity and reflex areas in reflexology: a functional magnetic resonance imaging study, *Neurosci Lett* 448(1):6–9, 2008.

National Collaborating Centre: *Routine care of the healthy pregnant woman. Clinical guideline*, 2008. Available online at www.nice.org.uk/nicemedia/pdf/CG62FullGuidelineCorrectedJune2008. Accessed January 2009.

Nilsson-Wikmar L, Harms-Ringdahl K, Pilo C, et al: back pain in women post–partum is not a unitary concept, *Physiother Res Int* 4(3):201–213, 1999.

Nurses and Midwives Act 2001/Nursing and Midwifery Order 2002: Statutory Document No. 159/02, Available online at www.gov.im/lib/docs/dhss/health/Sd159-02 Accessed January 2009.

NMC: Standards of conduct, performance and ethics for nurses and midwives, 2008. Available online at www.nmcuk.org/aFrameDisplay.aspx?DocumentID=3954. Accessed January 2009.

Ogai R, Yamane M, Matsumoto T, et al: Effects of petrissage massage on fatigue and exercise performance following intensive cycle pedaling, *Br J Sports Med* 42(10):534–538, 2008. Epub 2008 Apr 2.

O'Hara C: Challenging the "rules" of reflexology. In Mackereth P, Tiran D editors: *Clinical reflexology: a guide for health professionals*, Edinburgh, 2002, Elsevier, pp. 33–52.

O'Hara C, editor: *Core curriculum for reflexology in the United Kingdom*, London, 2006, Douglas Barry Publications.

O'Hara C: UK voluntary self-regulation by January 2008? *Clinical Reflexology News* Autumn 23:3–7, 2007.

O'Higgins M, St James Roberts I, Glover V: Postnatal depression and mother and infant outcomes after infant massage, *J Affect Disord* 109(1–2):189–192, 2008.

Oleson T, Flocco W: Randomized controlled study of premenstrual symptoms treated with ear, hand, and foot reflexology, *Obstet Gynecol* 82(6):906–911, 1993.

Omura Y: Accurate localization of organ representation areas on the feet & hands using the bi-digital O-ring test resonance phenomenon: its clinical implication in diagnosis & treatment – Part I, *Acupunct Electrother Res* 19 (2–3):153–190, 1994.

Osborne C: Supporting pregnancy with massage therapy, *Midwifery Today Int Midwife* 87 (Autumn): 20–21, 2008.

Osman JL: *Energy medicine. The scientific basis*, Edinburgh, 2000, Churchill Livingstone.

Park HS, Cho GY: Effects of foot reflexology on essential hypertension patients, *Taehan Kanho Hakhoe Chi* 34(5):739–750, 2004.

Panesar NS, Li CY, Rogers MS: Are thyroid hormones of hCG responsible for hyperemesis gravidarum? A matched paired study of pregnant Chinese women, *Acta Obstet Gynecol Scand* 80(6):519–524, 2001.

Papadopoulos EC, Khan SN: Piriformis syndrome and low back pain: a new classification and review of the literature, *Orthopaedic Clinics of North America* (35), (1):65–71, 2004. cited in Stone C: *Visceral and obstetric osteopathy*, Edinburgh, 2007, Churchill Livingstone.

Piquemal M: *Global effect of reflexology on blood flow,* 10th ICR International Conference, Amsterdam, September 2005.

Pistolese RA: The Webster Technique: a chiropractic technique with obstetric implications, *J Manipulative Physiol Ther* 25(6):E1–E9, 2002.

Popp FA: Principles of complementary medicine in terms of a suggested scientific basis.Indian, *J Exp Biol* 46(5):378–383, 2008.

Porter M, Bhattacharya S: Helping themselves to get pregnant: a qualitative longitudinal study on the information-seeking, *Hum Reprod* 23(3):567–572, 2008.

Pourghaznein T, Ghafari F: The effect of sole reflexology on severity of fatigue in pregnant women, *J Hayat* 12(4):5–12, 2006 (Persian). English abstract available online at journals.tums.ac.ir/abs. Accessed January 12, 2009.

Proctor ML, Hing W, Johnson TC, et al: Spinal manipulation for primary and secondary dysmenorrhoea, *Cochrane Database Syst Rev* (4): CD002119 2001.

Quattrin R, Zanini A, Buchini S, et al: Use of reflexology foot massage to reduce anxiety in hospitalized cancer patients in chemotherapy treatment: methodology and outcomes, *J Nurs Manag* 14(2):96–105, 2006.

Rabl M, Ahner R, Bitschnau M, et al: Acupuncture for cervical ripening and induction of labor at term – a randomized controlled trial, *Wien Klin Wochenschr* 113(23–24):942–946, 2001.

Raz I, Rosengarten Y, Carasso R: Correlation study between conventional medical diagnosis and the diagnosis by reflexology (non conventional), *Harefuah* 142(8–9):600–605, 646, 2003.

Reeson S: *Reflexology – the metamorphic technique*, 2006, Jamaica Gleaner June 19th.

Ricks S: Gentle touch of reflexology, *Positive Health* Issue 67, 2001. Available online at www.positivehealth.com/articleabstract.php?articleid=281. Accessed 3 March 2009.

Rubik B: The Biofield hypothesis: its biophysical basis and role in medicine, *J Altern Complement Med* 8(6):703–717, 2002.

Ruiz RJ, Avant KC: Effects of maternal prenatal stress on infant outcomes: a synthesis of the literature, *ANS Adv Nurs Sci* 28(4):345–355, 2005.

Sandman CA, Glynn L, Wadhwa PD, et al: Maternal hypothalamic-pituitary-adrenal disregulation during the third trimester influences human fetal responses, *Dev Neurosci* 25(1):41–49, 2003.

Sarno J: *The mind body prescription: healing the body, healing the pain*, New York, 1998, Warner Books.

Seers K, Crichton N, Martin J, et al: A randomised controlled trial to assess the effectiveness of a single session of nurse administered massage for short term relief of chronic non-malignant pain, *BMC Nurs* 4(7):10, 2008.

Selmer-Olsen T, Lydersen S, Mørkved S: Does acupuncture used in nulliparous women reduce time from prelabour rupture of membranes at term to active phase of labour? A randomised controlled trial, *Acta Obstet Gynecol Scand* 86(12):1447–1452, 2007.

Sharma JB, Sharma A, Bahadur A, et al: Oxidative stress markers and antioxidant levels in normal pregnancy and pre-eclampsia, *Int J Gynaecol Obstet* 94(1): 23–27, 2006.

Skouteris H, Wertheim EH, Rallis S, et al: Use of complementary and alternative medicines by a sample of Australian women during pregnancy, *Aust N Z J Obstet Gynaecol* 48(4):384–390, 2008.

Smith CA, Crowther CA, Collins CT, et al: Acupuncture to induce labor: a randomized controlled trial, *Obstet Gynecol* 112(5):1067–1074, 2008.

Solomon S: A review of mechanisms of response to pain therapy: why voodoo works, *Headache* 42(7):656–662, 2002.

Song RH, Kim DH: The effects of foot reflexion massage on sleep disturbance, depression disorder, and the physiological index of the elderly, *Taehan Kanho Hakhoe Chi* 36(1):15–24, 2006.

Stankiewicz M, Smith O, Alvino H, et al: The use of complementary medicine and therapies by patients attending a reproductive medicine unit in South Australia: A prospective survey, *Aust N Z J Obstet Gynaecol* 47(2):145–149, 2007.

Stephenson N, Dalton JA, Carlson J: The effect of foot reflexology on pain in patients with metastatic cancer, *Appl Nurs Res* 16(4):284–286, 2003.

Stephenson NL, Swanson M, Dalton J, et al: Partner-delivered reflexology: effects on cancer pain and anxiety, *Oncol Nurs Forum* 34(1):127–132, 2007.

Stone C: *Visceral and obstetric osteopathy*, Edinburgh, 2007, Elsevier.

Stormer C: *The language of the feet*, ed 2, London, 2007, Headline.

Sudmeier I, Bodner G, Egger I, et al: Changes of renal blood flow during organ-associated foot reflexology measured by color Doppler sonography, *Forsch Komplementarmed* 6(3):129–134, 1999.

Sugiura T, Horiguchi H, Sugahara K, et al: Heart rate and electroencephalogram changes caused by finger acupressure on planta pedis, *J Physiol Anthropol* 26(2): 257–259, 2007.

Tipping L: Practising in the neonatal area. In Mackereth P, Tiran D, editors: Clinical Reflexology, a guide for health professionals, Edinburgh, 2000, Elsevier, pp. 147–157.

Tipping L, Mackereth PA: A concept analysis: the effect of reflexology on homeostasis to establish and maintain lactation, *Complement Ther Nurs Midwifery* 6(4):189–198, 2000.

Tiran D: Breech presentation: increasing maternal choice, *Complement Ther Nurs Midwifery* 10(4):233–238, 2004a.

Tiran D: *Nausea and vomiting in pregnancy: an integrated approach to care*, Edinburgh, 2004b, Elsevier.

Tiran D, Chummun H: The physiological basis of reflexology and its use as a diagnostic tool, *Complement Ther Clin Pract* 11(1):58–64, 2005.

Tiran D: Complementary therapies in midwifery: a focus on moxibustion for breech presentation. In Marshall J, Raynor MD, editor: *Advancing midwifery skills*, Edinburgh, In press, Elsevier.

Tovey P: A single-blind trial of reflexology for irritable bowel syndrome, *Br J Gen Pract* 52(474):19–23, 2002.

Travell J, Simons T: *Myofascial pain & dysfunction: the trigger point manual*, Williams and Williams 1983, Baltimore. cited in Baldry PE: *Acupuncture, trigger points and musculoskeletal pain*, ed 3, Edinburgh, 2005, Elsevier.

van den Berg I, Bosch JL, Jacobs B, et al: Effectiveness of acupuncture-type interventions versus expectant management to correct breech presentation: a systematic review, *Complement Ther Med* 16(2):92–100, 2008.

Veith I: (translator) *The yellow emperor's classic of internal medicine*, Berkeley, 2002, University of California Press.

Wang MY, Tsai PS, Lee PH, et al: The efficacy of reflexology: systematic review, *J Adv Nurs* 62(5):512–520, 2008.

White AR, Williamson J, Hart A, et al: A blinded investigation into the accuracy of reflexology charts, *Complement Ther Med* 8(3):166–172, 2000.

Wilkinson S, Lockhart K, Gambles M, et al: Reflexology for symptom relief in patients with cancer, *Cancer Nurs* 31(5):354–360, 2008.

Williamson J: An introduction to precision reflexology, *Positive Health* Issue 29:1998. Available online at www.positivehealth. com/article–abstract.php?articleid=289. Accessed March 3, 2009.

Williamson J, White A, Hart A, Ernst E: Randomised controlled trial of reflexology for menopausal symptoms, *BJOG* 109(9):1050–1055, 2002.

Yang JH: The effects of foot reflexology on nausea, vomiting and fatigue of breast cancer patients undergoing chemotherapy, *Taehan Kanho Hakhoe Chi* 35(1):177–185, 2005.

Zhang CL: Acupuncture system and electromagnetic standing wave inside the body, *Nature* 17(4):52–62, 1995.

FURTHER READING

Reflexology and other complementary therapies

Booth L: *Vertical reflexology*, London, 2000, Piatkus.

Dougans I: *The new reflexology a unique blend of traditional Chinese medicine and Western reflexology practice for better health and healing*, New York, 2006, Marlowe and Co.

Dougans I: *Reflexology: The 5 elements and their 12 meridians – a unique approach*, London, 2007, Thorsons.

Mantle F, Tiran D: *An A–Z of complementary therapies for health professionals*, 2009, Edinburgh, Elsevier.

Tiran D, Mack S, editors: *Complementary therapies for pregnancy and childbirth*, ed 2, London, 2000, Baillière Tindall.

Tiran D, Mackereth P, editors: *Clinical reflexology: a guide for health professionals*, ed 2, Edinburgh, In press, Elsevier.

PREGNANCY AND CHILDBIRTH INFORMATION

Medforth J, Battersby S, Evans M, et al, editors: *Oxford handbook of midwifery*, Oxford, 2006, Oxford University Press.

Tiran D: *Teach yourself positive pregnancy*, London, 2008, Hodder Headline.

Tiran D: *Bailliere's midwives' dictionary*, ed 11, London, 2008, Elsevier.

References

Expectancy Ltd – Expectant Parents' Complementary Therapies Consultancy
Website: www.expectancy.co.uk

> Expectancy is the leading provider of professionally approved and university accredited courses on a variety of subjects related to the safe use of complementary therapies in pregnancy and childbirth. Courses include Caring for Pregnant Clients, Reflexology Techniques (RZT) for Maternity Care, the Diploma in Maternity Complementary Therapies (for midwives) and the Maternity Support Therapist (doula) programme (for therapists). Also provides information and advice for professionals and for mothers on the safe use of complementary therapies and natural remedies during the antenatal, intrapartum and postnatal periods, especially focusing on "morning sickness".

Federation of Antenatal Educators (FEDANT)
Website: www.fedant.org

> The Federation of Antenatal Educators (FEDANT) is the UK regulatory organisation for those providing antenatal education and preparation of expectant parents for birth and parenthood in order to protect the public. It provides a National Register of validated professionals within the field of antenatal education, including midwives, antenatal teachers, breastfeeding counsellors, doulas and complementary therapists. Also provides insurance cover for professionals.

Federation of Holistic Therapists (FHT)
Website: www.fht.org.uk

> The FHT is one of the leading professional organisations for complementary therapists, providing pre-registration and continuing professional education, indemnity insurance and adhering to standards of practice with a Code of Ethics and Professional Practice.

MIDIRS – Midwives' Information and Resource Service
Website: www.midirs.org

> MIDIRS is an educational charity, providing an international information resource relating to pregnancy, childbirth and the newborn, a database of contemporary research, an online enquiry and literature searching service, study days, "informed choice" leaflets for mothers and midwives and other activities.

National Center for Complementary and Alternative Medicine (NCCAM) database
Website: www.nccam.nih.gov/ camonpubmed

> This is a joint venture between the NCCAM and the National Library of Medicine (NLM) providing access to research abstracts from a variety of conventional and complementary medical and research databases, including MEDLINE and life science journals.

Reflexology Forum
Website: www.reflexologyforum.org

> The Reflexology Forum is the evolving UK regulatory body for reflexology, with a common set of standards for practice, a core educational curriculum for the preparation of practitioners and a remit to promote research, encourage professional development and the maintenance of high standards of practice to protect the public.

The Complementary and Natural Healthcare Council
Website: www.cnhc.org

> The CNHC is the emerging new body for voluntary self-regulation of complementary and alternative practitioners, including reflexologists, which opened to registration in January 2009.

Glossary of terms

Acupuncture aspect of traditional Chinese medicine based on the principle that the body has energy lines (meridians) running through it which link one part of the body to another. Application of acupuncture needles to disordered points aims to rebalance the energy flow and assist in achieving optimum health

Aetiology causes of disease

Anovulation absence of ovulation

Aromatherapy use of highly concentrated essential plant oils, administered by massage, in the bath, by inhalation, in compresses, douches, pessaries and creams, with therapeutic properties attributed to various chemicals

Blastocyst pregnancy about a week after conception which then reorganises and develops into the placenta and membranes and the fetus

Braxton Hicks contractions painless, irregular uterine contractions occurring during pregnancy which improve blood flow to the placenta and fetus

Calcaneum the heel bone

Cardiotocograph machine to monitor maternal and fetal progress and wellbeing in labour

Cephalopelvic disproportion condition in which the size of the fetal head is too large to traverse the mother's bony pelvis, requiring medical intervention in labour

Cervical incompetence failure of the cervix to remain closed and to keep the pregnancy within the uterus; a cause of second trimester miscarriage

Counternutation posterior movement (rocking or swaying) of the sacrum

Cuneiform bones three bones in the feet between the navicular and the metatarsal bones

Distal pertaining to being furthest from the midline, i.e. the distal surface of the foot is the outer edge

Dorsum upper surface of the foot

Episiotomy cut into the perineum during labour to enlarge the birth opening and allow space for the fetal head to emerge

Eutocia normal uterine action in labour

Fundus top, as in top of the uterus

Graafian follicle fluid-filled organism in the ovary from which the ovum (egg) develops

Grande multipara mother with five or more children

Homeostasis a physiological process of metabolic equilibrium

Hypertonic excessive tone in the muscles

Hypertrophy excessive growth of muscles or organs

Iatrogenic caused by medical treatment or interference

Idiopathic diseases or disorders of unknown cause

Intrapartum during labour

Involution a physiological process in which the uterus returns to its non-pregnant size, shape and position after delivery, over a period of 6–8 weeks

Iridology a diagnostic technique in which the iris of the eye is used as a complete map of the body, in the same way as the feet are used as the map in reflexology; it is not a therapeutic modality

Kyphosis abnormal backwards curvature (arching) of the upper spine

Lithotomy position the mother is positioned on her back with the thighs raised, knees supported and placed widely apart; used for forceps, ventouse extractions and breech deliveries

Lordosis abnormal forwards curvature (hollowing) of the spine, usually lower

LSCS lower segment Caesarean section

Medial pertaining to the middle, i.e. the medial aspect of the foot is the inner side

Metatarsals bones of the feet between the phalanges and the cuneiform bones

Moxibustion Chinese technique using a heat source (moxa stick) near an acupuncture point on the toes to attempt to turn a breech presentation to head-first

Myofascial trigger points hyperirritable spots in skeletal muscle, associated with palpable nodules in taut bands of muscle fibres, a common cause of pain

Navicular bone on the medial side of the foot, distal to the cuneiform bones

Nutation rocking or swaying

Phalanges the bones of the fingers and toes

Placental abruption separation of a normally situated placenta – causes painless bleeding

Placenta praevia abnormally situated placenta extending, in four grades, from the edge of the lower segment of the uterus, to the most serious grade, in which the complete placenta lies over the cervical opening; haemorrhage occurs as the cervix dilates and in grades 3 and 4, vaginal delivery is not possible

Plantar surface the sole of the foot

Pre-eclampsia a pregnancy-specific condition consisting of hypertension, oedema and protein in the urine which can lead to eclampsia in which the mother develops epileptic-type convulsions which can be fatal to both mother and baby

Puerperium postnatal period during which the mother's body returns to the non-pregnant state, usually lasting 6–8 weeks

Retroverted incarcerated gravid uterus condition occurring at about 14–16 weeks' gestation in which the abnormally positioned uterus (tilting backwards instead of forwards) is trapped by the bladder as it attempts to rise out of the pelvis into the abdominal cavity. This can cause sacculation of the uterus, spontaneous abortion and, most commonly, acute urinary retention due to over-stretching of the urethra

Salpingitis inflammation and infection in the fallopian tube(s)

Shiatsu a complementary therapy similar to acupressure, involving the application of thumb pressure to the acupuncture points on the body in order to restore and maintain homeostasis

Supine hypotension low blood pressure resulting from lying flat on the back – causes dizziness in the mother and may lead to fetal distress; women in late pregnancy should never be positioned flat on the back

Trendelenburg position position used for Caesarean section, in which the mother is supine but tilted to between 30° and 45° in order to take pressure off the inferior vena cava

Tsubo acupuncture point

Xiphisternum lower end of the sternum

For further definitions related to pregnancy and maternity care see:
Tiran D 2008 Bailliere's midwives' dictionary, 11th edn. Elsevier, Edinburgh

For further definitions related to complementary medicine see:
Mantle F, Tiran D 2009 A–Z of complementary and alternative medicine: a guide for health professionals. Elsevier, Edinburgh

Glossary of terms

Appendices

APPENDIX 1 SUGGESTED TREATMENT SEQUENCE FOR REFLEX ZONE THERAPY RELAXATION

The following is a guide to a possible routine which may be used for a relaxation treatment. The order of treatment may be changed or different/additional techniques may be incorporated; any specific techniques which are not appropriate should be omitted. Whichever routine the practitioner eventually develops as their own should ensure that the entire surface of both feet is covered with the "caterpillar crawling" movement; any identifiable zones requiring particular treatment are then worked with either sedating or stimulating movements.

The routine:

Make **contact** with feet from dorsal aspect

Stroking from knees to toes, dorsum
Bimanual stroking, down on dorsum, up on plantar surface

Relaxation point (solar plexus) – gently – plus **diaphragm** sweeping
Manipulation of bony parts of foot – ankle rotation, bimanual manipulation
   of top of foot
Advanced technique to relieve tension in the cervical vertebrae zones
   (see Appendix 2)
Heel holding and brisk heel rubbing

Cover the foot not being worked

Remember – each digit/foot has four surfaces – dorsum, plantar and two lateral
   aspects

Big toe – dorsum, sides, plantar surface – in "lawn-mower stripes"

Each of the **other toes**, all four surfaces

Dorsum of foot, from end of toes to inclination of the ankle – "caterpillar crawling" – use thumb, or one or more fingers, changing hands as necessary

Outer aspect of foot including around outer ankle bone

Inner aspect of foot including around inner ankle bone

Sole of foot – ball of the foot

Arch of the foot, *clockwise* direction

Heel of foot

Cover and **repeat** on other foot

Uncover both feet – finish with more relaxation stroking, heel work, manipulation
Solar plexus

Place both palms firmly over entire surface of plantar surface, remove slowly, finishing with fingertips coming off toes

Cover feet, stroking on top of towel, holding then release.

Reflex zone therapy sessions, even those performed merely for relaxation, should not exceed thirty minutes' duration during pregnancy and may frequently need to be shorter.

APPENDIX 2 MANIPULATIVE TECHNIQUES FOR STRUCTURAL REFLEX ZONE THERAPY

The nature of structural reflex zone therapy (RZT) means that it focuses on realigning the musculoskeletal system in order to restore homeostasis. The techniques employed are considerably more dynamic than some of the gentle techniques used in generic reflexology, and are akin to the manipulations used by osteopaths, but applied via the reflex zones of the feet rather than to the whole body. Structural RZT uses a forceful but not excessive degree of manipulation and the skill of the practitioner is to decide the amount of treatment that can be tolerated by the mother. These dynamic techniques also mean that the remainder of the treatment is likely to be shorter than normal, since not only will the mother be unable to tolerate a long session, but also, the anticipated outcome of the treatment is achieved sooner than with many generic systems of reflexology.

Manipulative techniques include holding and stretching of the heels, during which the practitioner applies slight traction with his/her palms cupped round the mother's two heels simultaneously. This is relaxing and particularly effective in labour as it extends that area of the feet corresponding to the pelvic area. Gentle rotation of the ankles, one at a time, in first one and then the other direction, stimulates pelvic circulation, aids pelvic lymphatic drainage and eases tension in the bony pelvis, particularly the pelvic brim.

Bimanually grasping that part of the foot corresponding to the ribcage, and using a firm "push–pull" movement to twist the sides of the feet, helps to release tension in the thoracic cavity. Another manipulation involves placing the two hands over the lateral (inner) edge of the foot so that all four fingers on each hand rest on the dorsum of the foot and the two thumbs rest on the plantar surface. A similar twisting movement is used so that the two hands rotate in opposite directions, thereby manipulating the areas corresponding to the ribcage and thoracic vertebrae. The movement should be controlled and employed only until the foot "cracks", signifying a release of tension in the thoracic area, or until the practitioner deems that no further manipulation is possible.

The advanced manipulative technique

The following advanced technique, used to stretch and ease the cervical vertebrae, should not be undertaken by the novice practitioner unless under supervision, as it is not without risk to the client. Over-vigorous rotation, lack of traction or failure to support the toe appropriately may lead to dislocation of the toe joints. The practitioner grips the big toe firmly at its base, between her second and third fingers with her palm uppermost and traction *must be applied* by the working hand before rotation commences. Her non-working hand *must* support the joint between the first (big) toe and the metatarsal with the medial edge of the bones in the practitioner's first finger placed over and above the bone. Each big toe should be *carefully and very slowly* rotated outwards. This means that the practitioner's right hand, working on the mother's left foot, will rotate clockwise, and her left hand, working on the mother's right foot, will rotate anti-clockwise so that the movement flows in a natural direction for each toe. It is vital not to over-extend the joints and to work only as far as the level of the client's comfort or until tension in the neck zones has been released: this is usually indicated by feeling the joints in the toe "give", and is often accompanied by a "crack" in the toe. The mother will often report that her neck feels more comfortable and is more mobile. Be aware that the mother can find this uncomfortable and some women do not like the sensations it induces. It can cause some women to feel sick especially if the practitioner's working fingers have not grasped the toe firmly enough and if they slide up and down the length of the toe, as this will be stimulating the reflex zone for the vagus nerve.

The advanced technique can be followed by applying tension-releasing traction to each of the other toes. The practitioner grasps the base of each toe with her dominant hand, using her thumb and forefinger. A short, sharp pull is applied to the base of the toe, which will elicit a "popping" sensation in those which are tense and/or rigid. The technique should be carried out on each of the other toes in turn, but should not be repeated if no reaction is forthcoming.

Condition	Zones	Precautions
Infertility, preconception care	General relaxation treatment Treat over several cycles Treat known causes where appropriate	Do NOT stimulate any specific zones unless it is appropriate to do so Treat both partners if possible Do NOT treat with reflex zone therapy (RZT) whilst woman is taking ovulatory stimulants, nor when fertilised embryos have been re-implanted into uterus, until pregnancy is well-established or menstruation occurs
Anxiety, tension, stress, preparation for labour; Tiredness, insomnia	General relaxation treatment; lungs, diaphragm sweeping, "solar plexus" to regulate breathing; stimulation and manipulation of shoulder zones and musculoskeletal system to relax; diverse sedation of heart zones to calm	Maximum duration 30–35 minutes Work gently if feet very tender
Nausea and vomiting	Light general relaxation treatment Manipulative techniques on musculoskeletal system zones Thyroid gland zone if appropriate Treat concomitant symptoms	Beware rapid profound reactions Care if h/o neck or back problems prior to pregnancy Avoid if on thyroid medication
Hypersalivation	Sedation of salivary gland zones Manipulation of head, neck, upper spine, rib zones Sedation of relevant teeth zones	
Headaches and migraine, neck pain	Symptomatic sedation of relevant head and neck zones Manipulation of spine zones Drainage of lymphatic zones if oedema	Be aware of causative factors, if known Caution if pre-eclampsia
Heartburn, indigestion	Sedation of oesophagus, cardiac sphincter Diaphragm sweeping; gentle stimulation of abdominal musculature zones Manipulation of thoracic spine zones	Do NOT sedate stomach zones
Constipation	Clockwise massage of arches of feet; stimulation of whole of gastrointestinal tract zone Stimulation of liver zone Stimulation of abdominal musculature zones Sedation of pelvic floor zones Manipulation of musculoskeletal zones	Always work in direction of peristalsis

Continued

Condition	Zones	Precautions
Haemorrhoids	Sedation of anal sphincter zones Stimulation of abdominal musculature and gastrointestinal zones	Always work in direction of peristalsis
Sinus congestion	Stimulation of zones for face, nose Drainage of lymphatic zones for head and neck Manipulation of zones for head, neck, ribs, shoulders, spine Very gentle stimulation of "solar plexus"	Observe reactions
Breech presentation	General relaxation treatment Manipulation of the zones for the musculoskeletal system Stimulation of Bladder 67 acupuncture point	Confirm presentation, listen to fetal heart prior to treatment Should not be performed before 34 weeks' gestation Do NOT treat if medical problems, previous or planned Caesarean section, raised BP, low lying placenta or antepartum bleeding
Backache, sciatica	Dynamic manipulation of spine, head, neck, rib cage, pelvis zones Diaphragm sweeping Sedation of both symptomatic and causative spine zones Sedation of sacroiliac joint, sciatic nerve and hip zones Stimulation of abdominal musculature zones	Ensure origin is musculoskeletal

Beware inadvertent stimulation of acupoints which may stimulate contractions – Bladder 60 & Spleen 6 |
| Symphysis pubis discomfort | Dynamic manipulation as above Sedation and sweeping of symphysis pubis zone Sedation of sacroiliac joint, sciatic nerve and hip zones | |
| Carpal tunnel syndrome | Sedation of hand/wrist zones Sweeping from hand to arm to shoulder zones Manipulation of shoulders, head, neck zones to ease pain Drainage of axillary and head/ neck lymphatic zones | Work towards heart |
| Oedema of ankles | Drainage of pelvic lymphatic zones Bimanual upwards leg massage Encourage mother to do wrist "wringing" Stimulation of renal tract zones | Caution if legs painful

Do NOT stimulate renal tract zones in presence of pre-eclampsia |

Copyright Expectancy 2008

APPENDIX 4 STRUCTURAL REFLEX ZONE THERAPY FOR LABOUR

Condition	Zones	Precautions
Anxiety, tension, stress, tiredness, especially in long labour	General relaxation to stimulate endorphins	Avoid uterus zones unless progress is slow
	Solar plexus including hand point	Adapt to mother's level and location of pain, anxiety, etc.
Fear, panic, "out of control"	Diaphragm "sweeping" and work over lung zones shoulder	
Pain relief in labour	zones to ease muscular tension	
	Ankle manipulation to facilitate pelvic outlet	
	Heel holding and cupping during contractions	
	Spine zones to regulate nerves – upper lumbar in first stage; lower lumbar in transition/second stage	
	Adrenal zone sedation to relieve panic, if appropriate	Avoid adrenal zones unless panic
	Vigorous ankle stimulation and/ or "wrist wringing" to ease pelvic congestion	Caution with own posture if mother mobile
Induction of labour, failure to progress, occipito-posterior position	Include all of above, as appropriate, plus:	*Therapists MUST discuss with midwife*
	Solar plexus and relaxation points	Do NOT stimulate uterus zone
	Stimulation of pituitary zones for oxytocin	
	Stimulation of sacroiliac joint and symphysis pubis zones to enlarge pelvic outlet	
	Acupressure stimulation to Spleen 6 points to increase and harmonise contractions	
	Acupressure stimulation to Bladder 60 point to encourage descent	*Bladder 60* – fetal head must flex before encouraging descent; avoid if cephalo-pelvic disproportion
Anterior lip of cervix, transition stage, slow progress in second stage	Include all techniques for relaxation, plus:	Do NOT use reflex zone therapy (RZT) in second stage if signs of fetal distress
	Pituitary stimulation if contractions slowed	
	Cervix zone stimulation to facilitate full dilatation	
	Pelvic joint zone stimulation to enlarge pelvic outlet	
	Sedation of solar plexus and heart zones to calm	
	Diaphragm sweeping and lungs to regulate breathing	
	Adrenal sedation (brief) if panic	

Continued

Condition	Zones	Precautions
Malpresentation/ position of fetus	Dynamic manipulation of musculoskeletal system Stimulation of sacroiliac joints Stimulation of Spleen 6 if uterine action poor	Do NOT stimulate uterus zone
	Stimulation of Bladder 60 once head is flexed	*Bladder 60* – fetal head must flex before encouraging descent, avoid if cephalo-pelvic disproportion
Hypertonic uterine action	Sedation of solar plexus to calm Sedation of adrenal zones to reduce impact of shock; general relaxation treatment if time allows	Brief, gentle work Do NOT stimulate uterus or pituitary gland zones
	Sedation of zones for abdominal musculature to suppress abdominal pain	Do *not* use these techniques if unsure of cause or effect
Retained placenta	Stimulation of pituitary zones to stimulate contraction if uterus not well contracted Sedation of solar plexus and abdominal zones, plus diaphragm sweeping to calm Bladder 60 acupoint stimulation to encourage descent ONLY if placenta separated Sedation of cervix zones ONLY if placenta separated and uterus well contracted	Do NOT perform these if h/o morbidly adherent placenta
Postpartum haemorrhage	Stimulation of pituitary zones to stimulate contraction of uterus Sedation of solar plexus and adrenal gland zones to reduce shock – ask partner to perform on hands	Use pituitary zone *only* if uterus fails to contract DO NOT stimulate uterus zone

Copyright Expectancy 2008

APPENDIX 5 STRUCTURAL REFLEX ZONE THERAPY FOR THE PUERPERIUM

Condition	Zones	Comments
Recovery from birth, anxiety, tiredness, insomnia	General relaxation treatment Stimulation OR sedation of adrenals, if appropriate Respiratory, adrenal, renal, gastro-intestinal and lymphatic systems Musculoskeletal system; gentle manipulation Abdominal wall Stimulation of liver to detoxify if drugs used in labour	Caution if P/N depression; avoid reflex zone therapy (RZT) if puerperal psychosis Caution if rectus sheath division or post-Caesarean Caution if still on medication
Headache, neck ache	Gentle manipulation of head, neck, spine, ribs, pelvis Sedation of specific points on head zone Manipulation of ribcage zones Gastrointestinal tract to aid detoxification	Avoid strong manipulation
Backache, sciatica	Gentle manipulation of head, neck, spine, ribs, pelvic bones and joints, knees Sedation of causative and symptomatic zones of spine Sedation of spine at site of epidural insertion Manipulation of shoulder girdle Sedation of hand if carpal tunnel Sweeping of symphysis pubis Generalised sedation of sciatic nerve Sedation of sacrum and coccyx Stimulation of abdominal muscles	Avoid strong manipulation Support metatarsal phalangeal joint Avoid if fracture Caution if post-Caesarean
Pain in legs, oedema	General relaxation treatment Sedation of knees Manipulation of musculoskeletal system Lymphatic drainage	Beware deep vein thrombosis
Perineal pain	Sedation of perineum, anus Lymphatic drainage in pelvis Stimulation of abdominal muscles Manipulation of musculoskeletal system	Care if Caesarean section
After Caesarean section	General relaxation treatment Stimulation of gastrointestinal tract Sedation of pelvic joints, hips Stimulation of respiratory tract Lymphatic drainage Stimulation of liver Gentle sedation of abdominal muscles	Caution if still on medication May be painful

Continued

Appendices

Condition	Zones	Comments
"After pains" with no apparent retained products	General relaxation treatment Sedation of "solar plexus" Diaphragm sweeping Sedation of uterus, tubes, ovaries Wrist wringing	Do NOT stimulate uterus
Heavy lochia, retained products of conception	As above, plus Pituitary stimulation Sedation of uterus and pelvic floor Stimulation of urinary system Manipulation of musculoskeletal system	Do NOT stimulate uterus Beware uterine infection or haemorrhage
Retention of urine	General relaxation treatment Stimulation of renal tract 3–5-minute treatments half hourly Ankle circling, brisk heel massage Wrist wringing Manipulation of musculoskeletal system Sedation of relevant spine and pelvic zones Stimulation of respiratory system	MUST be in direction of flow Beware urinary tract infection Work from coccyx to neck
Constipation, paralytic ileus after Caesarean section	Clockwise massage of arches of feet Stimulation of entire gastro-intestinal system Sedation of anal sphincter, perineum Stimulation of abdominal muscles Manipulation of musculoskeletal system, especially ribcage	Work clockwise over intestines Care if LSCS
Poor milk supply	Stimulation of pituitary Gentle massage of breast zones Self-massage of hand breast zone Manipulation of musculoskeletal system Advanced technique for neck Diaphragm sweeping Drainage of lymphatics in axilla and head and neck	
Engorgement of breasts	Light sedation of breast zones Drainage of lymphatics in axilla and head and neck Manipulation of musculoskeletal system Advanced technique for neck Diaphragm sweeping Stimulation of urinary system	Do NOT sedate breast zones
Suppression of lactation	General relaxation treatment Light sedation of breasts Drainage of axillary and head/neck lymphatics Stimulation of urinary system Stimulation of gastrointestinal tract "Solar plexus" sedation, holding	Do NOT stimulate breasts or pituitary

Index

E

F

Index

inter-vertebral discs, 14, 73
intestines zones, 78–9, 80
    constipation, 101
    haemorrhoids, 104
    lactation, 146
    postnatal care, 130, 143
    in pregnancy, 102–3
    see also large intestine; small intestine
intrauterine contraceptive device (IUD),
        41–2
in vitro fertilisation (IVF), 38
irritable bowel syndrome, 21, 86, 101

J

Japanese Ashitsubo, 63
jaw
    misalignment, nausea and vomiting, 92
    zone
        hypersalivation, 96
        location, 96

K

kidney(s)
    calculi, 41, 69
    and psoas muscle, 138
    in the puerperium, 138–42
    zone, 77, 80
        oedema, 109
        postnatal care, 140
        sinus congestion, 110
knees, 59, 75, 132, 133
kyphosis, 14, 18

L

labour, 44, 113–25, 163–4
    abnormal, 45
    acceleration, 117–23, 163
    estimation of onset, 116–17
    first stage, 44
    induction, 44, 117–23, 163
        case study, 122–3
        relevant reflexology treatment, 118–22
        structural physiology and aetiology,
            117–18
    intervention in, 128
    pain relief in, 114–16
    prediction, 70
    preterm, 43
    problems in, 24
    third stage, 123–5
lacrimal duct, 71
lactation, 22, 143–6
    hormones, 128
    suppression, 166

lactic acid crystals, 49
large intestine, 78–9, 142
Large Intestine 4 acupoint, 120
legal issues, 26–8
lesser omentum, 142
let down reflex, 143, 145
light-headedness after treatment, 55
lighting, 31–2
Likert scale, 36
limb fractures, 17
limbic system, 129
limb length discrepancy, 16
lithotomy position, 133
liver, 59
    zone, 80
        constipation, 101
        haemorrhoids, 104
        postnatal care, 130
lochia, 134, 166
lordosis, 13, 14, 18
lower limbs
    oedema, 108
    pain, postnatal, 165
    zones, 75
lumbar spine, 14, 73
lungs zone, 81–2
    lactation, 144
    palpitations, 90
    in the puerperium, 140
lymphatic drainage, 22
    head and neck, 71
    oedema, 108–9
    postnatal care, 130, 137
    sinus congestion, 110
lymphatic system
    axillary, 67–8, 76
    head and neck, 71, 76
    inflammation, 41
    pelvic, 67, 76
    zones, 76

M

mammary glands, 67–8
    see also breasts
manipulation, 52, 53, 159–60
Marquardt, Hanne, 2
Marquardt reflex zone therapy, 20
massage, 4–5, 24, 49, 52
    vs. reflexology, 4, 20
mastitis, 146
mechanoreceptors, 4
medial umbilical ligaments, 138
medication, 44
Meissner's corpuscles, 4
menstrual cycle, 64–5, 70–1
meridian reflexology, 6–7, 8
meridians of acupuncture, 6–7, 119, 121

Index

Q

R

S

schizophrenia, 42
Schumann resonance, 6
sciatica
  postnatal, 165
  in pregnancy, 162
  relevant reflexology treatment, 106–7
  structural physiology and aetiology, 104–6
sciatic nerve, 75, 106
scoliosis, 14
sedation, 50–1, 53
  pituitary point, 63–4
  stress/anxiety, 90
  uterus zone, 65
sensory nerve receptors, skin, 4
serotonin, 3
sham reflexology, 4–5
shiatsu (acupressure), 24, 28
shoulder zones, 73–4
  carpal tunnel syndrome, 108
  lactation, 144
  postnatal care, 132, 133
sinus congestion, 110, 162
skin
  elasticity, 48
  irregularities, foot, 48
  sensory nerve receptors, 4
skull vault, 71
small intestine, 78–9, 80, 142
SMART Ayurvedic Reflexology, 9
solar plexus, 59, 60–2
  labour, 114, 115–16
  lactation, 146
  locating, 61
  nausea and vomiting, 93
  overstimulation, 62
  postnatal care, 130, 135
  sinus congestion, 110
  stress/anxiety, 89–90, 90–1
somatic pain, 115
sperm abnormalities, 85
spinal reflexology, 10
spinal twist, 133
spine
  bone, 13–14
  changes in pregnancy, 18–19
  curves, 13, 14
  lumbar, 14
  mal-adaptation, 13
  misalignment
    breech presentation, 111
    postnatal, 131, 132
  movement, 14–15
  nerve damage, 139
  structural reflex zone therapy (RZT), 13–15
  thoracic, 14
  zones, 72–3
    haemorrhoids, 104
    labour, 116
    lactation, 144

nausea and vomiting, 94
  in the puerperium, 130, 132, 133, 137, 140
  stress/anxiety, 90
Spleen 6 acupoint, 120–1, 122, 124
spleen zone, 76
Stathis Method of Ayurvedic Reflex Therapy (SMART), 9
sternocleidomastoid tension, 129
stimulants, 53
stimulation, 50, 51, 53
  pituitary point, 63–4
  uterus zone, 65
stomach zone, 78, 100
stress, 3, 20, 88–91
  after childbirth, 129
  diaphragm sweeping, 62
  effect on posture, 16
  patterns manifested in feet, 4
  in pregnancy, 161
  relevant reflexology treatment, 89–91
  structural physiology and aetiology, 88–9
stress hormones, 86, 89
  labour, 115
  and touch, 3
  see also specific hormone
structural adaptation, 15–17
sub-fertility see infertility
swayback posture, 18
sweeping, 52
  see also diaphragm, sweeping
sympathetic nervous system, 129
symphysis pubis, 15
  discomfort
    in pregnancy, 162
    relevant reflexology treatment, 106–7
    structural physiology and aetiology, 104–6
  zones, 74, 132, 133, 140, 143
synergistic reflexology, 8
systematic reviews, 21

T

teeth zones, 71–2
temporomandibular joint pain, 129
tenderness, 54
tension, 47
  after childbirth, 129
  in labour, 163
  postnatal, 131
  in pregnancy, 161
therapeutic relationship, 4–5
thoracic nerves, 142
thoracic spine, 14
  zones, 72–3
    lactation, 144, 146
    postnatal care, 133

Printed in the United States
By Bookmasters